GET CONTROL OF SUGAR NOW!

For more information on Paul McKenna and his books,
see his website at www.paulmckenna.com

www.**penguin**.co.uk

Also by Paul McKenna

INSTANT INFLUENCE AND CHARISMA

FREEDOM FROM EMOTIONAL EATING

THE HYPNOTIC GASTRIC BAND

I CAN MAKE YOU SMARTER

I CAN MAKE YOU HAPPY

I CAN MAKE YOU THIN

I CAN MAKE YOU THIN: 90-DAY SUCCESS JOURNAL

I CAN MAKE YOU THIN: LOVE FOOD, LOSE WEIGHT! (illustrated)

CONTROL STRESS

I CAN MAKE YOU SLEEP

I CAN MAKE YOU RICH

QUIT SMOKING TODAY

INSTANT CONFIDENCE

CHANGE YOUR LIFE IN SEVEN DAYS

I CAN MEND YOUR BROKEN HEART (with Hugh Willbourn)

THE HYPNOTIC WORLD OF PAUL McKENNA

GET CONTROL OF SUGAR NOW!

•

PAUL McKENNA PH.D.

EDITED BY HUGH WILLBOURN PH.D.

BANTAM PRESS

LONDON · TORONTO · SYDNEY · AUCKLAND · JOHANNESBURG

TRANSWORLD PUBLISHERS
61–63 Uxbridge Road, London W5 5SA
www.penguin.co.uk

Transworld is part of the Penguin Random House group of companies
whose addresses can be found at global.penguinrandomhouse.com

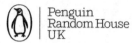

First published in Great Britain in 2016 by Bantam Press
an imprint of Transworld Publishers

A CIP catalogue record for this book
is available from the British Library.

ISBN 9780593075685

Typeset in 11/17pt Palatino by Julia Lloyd Design
Printed and bound by Clays Ltd, Bungay, Suffolk

Penguin Random House is committed to a sustainable
future for our business, our readers and our planet. This book
is made from Forest Stewardship Council® certified paper.

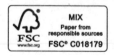

1 3 5 7 9 10 8 6 4 2

CONTENTS

ACKNOWLEDGEMENTS

I want to acknowledge the remarkable scientists and others who have worked for so many years in the face of considerable opposition to reveal the true nature of sugar and the dangers it represents.

The late Professor Yudkin of Queen Elizabeth College, London was a great man who saw fifty years ago what sugar could do. If governments and scientists had listened to him then, we would not be facing such a crisis of disease and obesity now.

In the present day, the leading figure in the fight against sugar is the tireless Dr Robert Lustig of the University of California, San Francisco. His book *Fat Chance* is a very readable introduction to the scientific research and a fact-filled study of the social and medical environment.

Many, many other scientists, doctors, journalists, writers and film-makers have been working to expose the truth about sugar and I offer my sincere thanks and respect to them all. Their work has shown that we absolutely must reduce sugar consumption now.

I hope this book will help people make the changes we now know are vital.

My thanks to all the people who assisted me in the immense amount of effort it has taken to produce this book, including Dr Hugh Willbourn, whose dedication, tireless research and work ethic are exceptional, my wife Kate McKenna, Doug Young, Janine Giovanni, Alex Tuppen, Jason Fraser, Dr Ronald Ruden, Mike Osborne and Mari Roberts.

READ THIS FIRST!

Inside the cover of this book is a CD. It contains powerful techniques that are a vital part of the system of change in this book. Please use it only as instructed.

The first track is the relaxing, eyes-closed, mind-programming process. You must listen to it only in a place where you can safely be unaware of the outside world and remain undisturbed for twenty-five minutes. Do not use it while driving or operating machinery.

On the following tracks I will talk you through the techniques in this system, so that you can listen and do them yourself at the same time.

Please use the CD every day for the first seven days, and at least once a week thereafter. You can use it more often if you like.

You can also download the audio files by visiting **www.paulmckenna.com/downloads** and entering the code **4TL39GY9X**.

WELCOME

•

THE HEALTHIEST DECISION OF YOUR LIFE

THE HEALTHIEST DECISION OF YOUR LIFE

Welcome! I believe this is the most important book I have ever written. A bold statement, I know, but one I have never made before in over twenty years of writing books. As you use this book you will not only improve your own health, you will be part of a revolution. For years my medical friends had been telling me that sugar is bad and, like most people, I dismissed their talk as just the latest health fad or another scare story. I thought it wasn't that important. How wrong was I.

By the time you finish this book, you, like me, will have changed what you eat and transformed your understanding of sugar. The tipping point came for me at the beginning of a long day's work with my good friend Dr Ronald Ruden. I poured a large cup of coffee and I said, 'I need some sugar to get me through this. Where's the sugar?'

Ron replied, 'There's no sugar in this house. And there never will be.'

'Hang on,' I said. 'I know it's a bit fattening, but you must have some somewhere. A couple of spoonfuls can't be that bad.'

Ron was appalled. 'Do you know what that stuff does to you?' he asked.

I shrugged because, in truth, at that point I didn't.

'Sugar,' said Ron, 'is the most dangerous drug in the world.'

Ron is a medical nutritionist and one of the most respected doctors in America. He explained how the world has been conned. I spent the next thirty minutes in shock as he listed all the medical and psychological damage that sugar can do. I was determined to understand why sugar is so dangerous. I could scarcely believe what I found.

The evidence is overwhelming

I discovered research that shows unequivocally that sugar is implicated in four of the top five causes of premature death in the UK. Sugar raises the risk of heart attacks, strokes and hypertension. The more sugar people eat, the higher their risk of diabetes. In the UK alone there are twenty amputations a day as a result of diabetes. Studies have shown that sugar accelerates the growth of cancers. Sugar has been implicated in both depression and dementia. A famous scientific study found that sugar was more addictive than cocaine.

If sugar was discovered today it would be banned.

Sugar has a unique way of bypassing the body's defences, and behind the innocent façade of sweetness sugar is slowly poisoning us. It is the single most deadly element of the global industrial diet. And it is everywhere. It is inserted into more than 75 per cent of all the foodstuffs in your local supermarket.

I have written many books about personal development, hypnosis and self-improvement but I have never written a book like this before. My intention was to write a simple book to help people. I found myself exploring a biological mystery, a political thriller and a terrifying tale of misdirection, bad science and foul play.

Some of what you are about to read will fly in the face of what people believe is common sense and what you have been told by doctors, teachers and scientists – but amazingly the entire establishment has been misled for over thirty years. I found it hard to believe how so much bad science had been allowed to go unchallenged for so long. However, my research and that of all my team left no doubt.

You may be shocked and even frightened by what you learn in this book, but the good news is I would not have written it if I didn't have a solution. As you read this book from cover to cover and follow all my instructions completely, you will reduce your sugar consumption and massively reduce your risk of heart disease, diabetes, obesity and many other diseases, even cancer.

Follow my instructions and join me in a healthier, happier and longer life.

1
.

YOUR LIFE WILL CHANGE FOR THE BETTER NOW

YOUR LIFE WILL CHANGE FOR THE BETTER NOW

I started with a mission and I've ended up on a crusade. I discovered that sugar is more than a matter of personal taste. I have always believed that diets are a con and I still believe that, along with the leading doctors and researchers in the field. But there is one thing, just one single, 'natural' additive, against which our bodies and our minds are defenceless. It derails the beautifully balanced system that keeps us well nourished and healthy. That additive is sugar. The amount varies from person to person but for each of us there is a tipping point. When we eat more than a certain amount of sugar we lose control of our bodies and we corrupt the natural system that keeps us fit and healthy.

My mission is to help you regain that control, and as you do so with every page you turn and every technique you use, you will find that not just your health but other parts of your life improve too. It is not necessary to stop consuming sugar completely. You will reach a point where you can enjoy it in safe amounts and also feel satisfied without it.

My crusade is to help you rescue yourself and your family before you eat yourselves to a slow and painful death. You may think I am being melodramatic here. In fact, it is impossible to exaggerate the dangers of sugar personally, nationally and globally. However, even though the reality of how sugar has invaded our food supply is terrifying, remember this book also contains your personal escape route.

Every nation in the world needs to reduce their sugar consumption substantially and rapidly. Diseases caused by chronic sugar consumption are making people sick all over the globe. In the UK they are bankrupting the National Health Service. In the USA, Medicare is predicted to go bust within seven years. Sugar doesn't kill people quickly like cyanide. Sugar mostly kills people very slowly, painfully and very, very expensively.

The world simply cannot afford to continue like this.

People say 'sugar is just a bit naughty'

Like most people, at first I just had a vague idea that too much sugar was not very good for you. I grew up believing that sugar was a bit naughty but if I brushed my teeth properly I would be all right. I later understood that sugar was fattening so I shouldn't eat too much but that was the limit of my knowledge. I had absolutely no idea of the menace that is hidden in sugar.

The appearance of innocence

Sugar has an image of innocence. It is pure and white and sweet. We like sweetness so much that we use 'sweet' to mean kind, touching, cute, attractive, adorable and lovable. 'Sugar', 'Sweetheart' and 'Honey' are the words we use for our loved ones. Languages all over the world are saturated with positive associations to sugar. Sweet is a word all about goodness. There are thousands of songs about sugar and candy and love.

Sweetness is the world's favourite taste. In different countries people eat different sorts of food. What some like, others hate. Some people like sour fermented cabbage and some people hate it. Some people like fish sauce, other people hate it. But everyone loves sugar. Cakes and cookies, desserts and puddings, colas, soft drinks and juices sell like hot cakes all over the world. We even use the simile 'hot cakes' to describe items selling extremely fast.

How come such deliciousness, a symbol of beauty, love, hope and joy is now irrefutably linked to killer diseases, disability, depression and a worldwide medical disaster? How did sugar lose its innocence?

Sugar is the stuff of treats and sweets and children's birthday parties. It seems too grotesque that the little rewards we give our children and the way we cheer ourselves up are killing us.

We all know that people with a sweet tooth are often a little on the tubby side, but surely it can't be that bad? Surely sweet little sugar can't cause dementia, amputations, blindness, strokes and heart attacks? The more I found out, the more incredible it seemed.

I just could not believe sugar could be deadly. Sugar is sweet, it's tasty, it makes you feel good and makes food taste better. How could it possibly be killing us? No one eats one spoonful of sugar and falls down dead. So how can it be so dangerous?

Why the sudden rise in obesity?

The glaringly obvious sign of chronic ill-health and food mismanagement is the global epidemic of obesity. Worldwide, obesity has doubled since 1980. In the UK, two-thirds of adults and a quarter of children between two and ten years old are overweight or obese. But no one in power is willing to state the cause. All the governments and advisory bodies and food manufacturers want to blame individuals. They say people should diet. They say people should eat less and exercise more. They all want to pretend that somehow in just thirty years two-thirds of the population have become greedy and lazy to a degree that is unprecedented in world history.

The medical evidence tells a very different story. People get fat because they eat too much, and they eat too much because they have lost control of their appetite. Sugar overturns the natural feelings of hunger and fullness. Sugar takes over people's appetite. The culprit is sugar.

Obesity doesn't kill anyone, but people die from the diseases that go with obesity or from damage caused by the stress it puts on the body. I don't believe people choose to put themselves in harm's way like that. Obesity is not a free, sane, healthy choice.

I know from the tens of thousands of overweight people with whom I have worked that they did not choose to be obese. It happened to them, because they found they couldn't stop eating. The food they ate was overwhelmingly processed food, manufactured food, fast food and junk food, and it is all rammed full of sugar.

Diet clubs make it far, far worse

Dieting is a recipe for disaster. Going to a diet club makes people lose weight in the short-term but then they put it all back on, and more, in the long-term. When people eat less, their body acts as though there is a famine and goes into survival mode, slows down the metabolism and begins to store energy as fat. As soon as dieters stop rigidly controlling their food, they eat more than before to store up energy for the next famine. That's why 70 per cent of people on any diet end up heavier than when they started. And because many people go on diet after diet after diet, and each time they have a 70 per cent chance of gaining weight, pretty soon almost all dieters end up fatter.

Diet clubs sell special, expensive 'low-fat' diet foods that are laced with sugar and they just make the situation worse, because the dieters end up even hungrier. The diet clubs make money by selling expensive diet foods and meal substitutes. They make even more money because they don't work. If diet clubs worked, by now they would all have shut up shop because all their members would be thin and would be walking adverts for the success of the clubs.

Sugar propaganda

The battlefield is not the restaurant, the kitchen or the supermarket. Those are the places where you will see the evidence of your victory, but the key lies elsewhere.

The real battlefield is in your mind.

Sugar and the forces that push it have invaded your brain physically and psychologically. Your brain chemistry has been changed by sugar. At the same time your imagination has been polluted by years and years of advertising and subliminal influences so that the most personal celebrations and most joyful events have been subverted to sell you manufactured, preserved, packaged, sweetened poison.

Large corporations seize every opportunity to sell more sugar and they choose to ignore the huge body of evidence that shows it is dangerous. Experts who have spoken out against sugar have been marginalized or silenced by the powerful elite of corporate industry interests, through the politicians they support and their well-funded scientific friends.

Even though sugar is more dangerous than cigarettes, there are no public health warnings on products containing sugar. There should be a notice on every product that contains sugar:

PUBLIC HEALTH WARNING

SUGAR IS HIGHLY DANGEROUS

Sugar is implicated in four of the top five causes of premature death in the United Kingdom

REDUCE YOUR SUGAR CONSUMPTION NOW

High sugar

There is a vast amount of sugar in soft drinks, cereals and even in savoury sauces. There is excessive sugar in supposedly healthy products like flavoured yoghurts, fruit juice, vitamin water and granola bars. As you read this book you will find out how to prevent sabotage by sugar, how to stay healthy and enjoy everything you eat.

Sugar lies

I fully expect the sugar industry and their paid scientists to attack me. They will say that 'all calories count' and it is the responsibility of the consumer to count calories. The theory of calorie-counting has been completely discredited. For thousands of years people naturally controlled their weight by stopping eating when they were full. No one counted calories. They were guided by their own bodies. Now their guidance system has been corrupted by sugar. Calorie-counting is a con invented by the diet industry and it doesn't work.

The body is not like a warehouse that stores calories and sends them back out again. You cannot swap one calorie for another. The body transforms all your food into a myriad of different chemicals and, as we shall see, it treats sugar differently from any other food.

The sugar industry will say that sugar is a useful nutrient and can form part of a balanced diet. The truth is sugar contains nothing essential at all, and it is difficult to have a 'balanced' diet when 75 per cent of all the foods in the shops have added sugar. If you never ate another gram of sugar in your life your body would get everything you need from other foods, and furthermore you would automatically be in the healthiest 20 per cent of the population.

Sugar is totally unnecessary.

The sugar industry will say people should take more exercise, and it is their own fault they are fat. Exercise is very good for you, but it is not an efficient way to lose weight. The more you exercise, the more you want to eat, because your body refuels and builds muscle to meet the demands of exercise. That is very healthy, but it won't make up for eating or drinking too much sugar. You would have to ride a bicycle for five miles to burn off the calories in just one can of soda. People don't gain weight because they don't do exercise – they don't do exercise because they have gained weight. They gained weight eating sugar.

You will find that after you lose weight you will want to do something energetic. Your muscles are made for moving and, once they are not exhausted from carrying around too much fat, you will enjoy it. Human beings love to enjoy their bodies.

You do not have to go the gym. Ironically, the massive expansion of the gym business is also fuelled by the obesity epidemic, but only the most obsessed gym rats actually benefit. Most people join in January and quit before the end of February because it doesn't work. Exercise can make you fit and healthy and it is a very good thing indeed. It is just a very inefficient way to lose weight.

The answer is easier than you think

By the time you finish this book I want you to know the truth. Sugar is too dangerous to be ignored. There is irrefutable science that sugar kills. I want you to know about it so you will no longer be deceived by the corporations who want you to keep buying. You will be free and back in control of your food.

We now have the psychological technology to reverse the distortions created by sugar and restore the landscape of your brain to a healthy, bright, balanced freedom. We can cleanse your mind and set your highest aspirations free from cynical exploitation so you can truly enjoy life to the full, in all its delicious sensory detail.

All you have to do is to read this book, cover to cover, and use the techniques exactly as directed.

When we have finished, your life will be fuller, richer and healthier and you will even be able to enjoy sugar properly again. You will be able to experience it without any guilt as the special, rare, delicious treat it once was.

Silent, slow and deadly

Sugar is behind all the biggest health problems of the twenty-first century. Sugar's deadly secret is that it is a slow-motion poison. Sugar is remorseless. Sugar creeps up softly, sweetly, without warning and little by little by little it pollutes the bloodstream, corrodes the liver and blocks the arteries. Sugar can take decades to kill. But sugar can make life painful and difficult long before death. Some people die from a fatal heart attack out of the blue. Others have diabetes, strokes or heart disease and live for years with painful or limiting disabilities.

It is not just about weight

We are all aware now of the outrageous increase in obesity in the last thirty years. One in four Britons and one in three US citizens are now obese – not just overweight, obese. But obesity is just one of the problems caused by sugar and it is not even the worst. Eighty per cent of obese people and 40 per cent of people who are not obese or overweight have a syndrome caused by sugar that is the precursor to heart disease, strokes and diabetes. People can look perfectly healthy on the outside and have no sign of sickness at all until it is far, far too late.

It is not just bad luck

I don't want to frighten you too much. But I do want to frighten you enough so that you take this situation seriously. The point is that the massive rise in heart disease, diabetes, cancer and dementia in the last thirty years is not just bad luck. It is not an accident. It is not a fluke. It is caused by sugar and it is entirely preventable. We can all live heathier, happier, longer lives and we can save our nations a fortune in healthcare costs if we all do just one thing: reduce our sugar consumption. Read on and find out how.

This is not a diet

There are no recipes or meal plans in this book. I don't have any expensive wonder foods to sell you. There are plenty of books with low-sugar recipes and you can find them and use them as much as you want. You don't need expensive, branded additives and you don't need to count calories or stick to fancy diets. You just need to regain control of your own appetite and let your taste buds guide you to ordinary, healthy, fresh food.

This book and CD form a unique system. It doesn't just tell you what you need to do. It helps you to actually do it. Together we will change your behaviour and your choices so that you massively reduce your intake of sugar and never feel like you are missing out.

This programme will take you all the way to the state in which you will feel fitter, lighter, healthier and happier than you ever did when you were unconsciously consuming kilos of sugar every year.

As you get more control of your appetite, you will have all you need to make your own choices for delicious food and to stay healthy. I want you to be free to choose what to eat and drink every day to keep yourself healthy and happy. There are a million different ways to get that right. But first of all you have to be in full possession of all the wisdom and guidance of your body.

Now is the time to change

As you use the system in this book you will change the way you eat. This book contains a psychological system that will restore your control over your sugar consumption. You will consume less sugar. That means you will eat and drink fewer products with added sugar. However, you will enjoy your food differently. You will eliminate cravings and re-establish a cycle of genuine hunger followed by genuine satisfaction.

Some of the change will happen in how you buy food. You will eat more protein and vegetables and lose weight too, but you don't have to think about it. All you need to do is follow my instructions until your appetite has recalibrated, and then trust your instincts. You may end up cooking your own food more often, but it is not necessary. You don't need to be a master chef.

You do not need to completely eliminate sugar from your diet, but you will be free to do so if you wish. You will recalibrate your own natural system so that you are able to eat sugar in safe and enjoyable quantities.

THE POWER OF THIS SYSTEM

This book is a system with three elements:

- **Essential information**
- **Powerful techniques**
- **Mind-programming**

Essential Information

We have never had access to so much information, nor been exposed to so much advertising. Unfortunately, much of what you can access on the internet is inaccurate, incomplete or unhelpful. Some is downright misleading. As we will see in the next chapter, even scientific research now has to be approached cautiously. Corporate interests and academic egos can stand in the way of a truly impartial approach. When there are billions to be made and status is at stake, no one wants to acknowledge inconvenient truths.

You need to know a few facts about sugar that food manufacturers don't want you know. I'm assuming you don't have a degree in biochemistry. You don't need it. The scientific evidence is presented simply here so that you understand what is happening, why you need to change it, and how you will change it.

Powerful techniques

My expertise is in psychology and human behaviour. All the excellent scientists working on the metabolism of sugar have shown us its dangers. My job here is to present the evidence in an easy-to-understand way and, more importantly, to program your mind so that it will reduce your sugar intake and so that you and your family get safe.

People eat sugar because it is easy, convenient and tasty. They like it. As you get control of sugar, I want you to enjoy life just as much as the sugar-eaters, but to stay healthy so you enjoy it for longer. I'm not here to deprive you of anything. I want you to know that when you put in the effort to use the techniques I am showing you, you can enjoy food and drink just as much, and even more, and you will also be rewarded with years of health and happiness.

I have developed these techniques over many years in many different contexts and each year I improve them. The system in this book has been created from years of work changing behaviour around food. I have included the most powerful techniques in my armoury and specially refined them for this task.

Now that we know the truth about sugar, we can apply these techniques and strategies to put you back in control. I have just one warning: I can't do the techniques for you. You have to do them. Commit to following this programme. When you commit, you benefit immediately and you can track your progress in the journal.

We use the first seven days to recalibrate your hormonal signalling system and your psychological default settings. You will perceive a re-patterning of your thoughts and behaviours. During the following thirty days you will track the long-term impact of those changes and cement them into your daily life. During those thirty days you will prove to yourself the value of this programme. I'm asking you to put in these thirty-seven days of effort now to set yourself up to be healthier and happier for the rest of your life.

Mind-programming

There are many types of mind-programming. Athletes call it 'mental rehearsal', where they imagine winning over and over again. Einstein called it 'thought experiments', in which he visualized how the universe could work. Modern psychologists use techniques like hypnosis, which is a concentrated form of imagination. I have drawn on all these techniques to create a safe yet extremely powerful programme to focus your unconscious mind to support you as you reduce your use of sugar.

When you use the mind-programming technique on the CD, I will program your unconscious mind. Your unconscious mind will use the facts about the metabolism of sugar to recalibrate your responses and restore your control over your appetite.

It doesn't matter whether you listen with your conscious mind or not. You can drift or dream and you can even fall asleep as you listen and the process will work fine. Your unconscious will hear all you need to change your sensitivity and response to sugar so that you become free of any habit or sugar cravings and are free to eat as little sugar as is right for you.

THE CD

On the CD I will talk you through the techniques in the book. The first track is the relaxing, eyes-closed, mind-programming process. You must listen to it only in a place where you can safely be unaware of the outside world and remain undisturbed for twenty-five minutes. Do not use it while driving or operating machinery.

You do not have to make any special effort when you are listening to the mind-programming process. Just put the CD on and let your unconscious mind hear what it needs to hear.

After the mind-programming, I will take you through each of these psychological techniques, one step at a time: The Craving Buster, Program Your Mind for a Healthy Future, The Swish, Instant Feel Good and Havening.

Please use the CD every day for the first seven days, and at least once a week thereafter. You can use it more often if you like. The book and CD together will help you make exactly the changes you need.

THE POWER OF JOURNALING

I would like you to keep a very short journal at the back of this book in which you note the techniques you use and the changes you make, one day at a time.

Journaling has been shown to help people stay on track with behavioural change. As Oprah Winfrey said, 'Journaling changed my life.'

Modern science has shown: 'What gets measured gets done.' A journal is like reporting to yourself. It supports emotional balance and awareness of your achievement. As you keep track of the changes you make, you will find it easier and easier to keep going in the right direction and feel in control.

Right now I'd like you to make a note of your normal consumption of sugar. It does not have to be a perfect list, and you don't need to hunt down every last gram of sugar. You may find out later that some of the things you drink or eat contain far more sugar than you realize. That doesn't matter now, you can add them to the list later. Just make a note now of the sugar you normally eat or drink.

Next, highlight where and when you feel you are consuming too much sugar. When you look back on this list in a few weeks' time, you will be amazed at your own success.

So grab a pen and turn to page 153 now. Make sure you complete that first day of the journal now, then come back here and read on.

START THE CHANGE NOW

Now that you have a note of where you started, it is time to begin the journey to freedom. We will start by making sure that you are free of sugar cravings.

Sugar cravings, like emotional eating, are not real hunger. True hunger is the feeling of an empty stomach. In this food-filled world with three meals a day and snacks available all around us all the time, many of us no longer know what it is like to have an empty stomach. True hunger is satisfied by good nourishment. When you are properly hungry, a balanced meal will appear more attractive to you than biscuits or a cake.

First of all, we must find out whether you are experiencing hunger, thirst or cravings. Next time you think you want to eat or drink something specifically containing sugar, ask yourself:

Am I really hungry?

Forget your thoughts for a second and check in with the *feeling* in your stomach. Does it feel empty?

If the answer is no, it is a craving, so use the Craving Buster at the end of this chapter.

If the answer is yes, ask the next question:

Will it satisfy my hunger if I eat something that is not sugary?

If the answer is yes, go ahead and eat something that is not sugary. Your problem is solved!

If the answer is no, or you are even a bit unsure, there is an element of craving, so use the Craving Buster at the end of this chapter.

Eliminate cravings

About ten years ago, a famous British actress asked me if I could help her to control her chocolate habit. She was eating about eight bars a day. She was not an ounce overweight but she was worried that it might be affecting her health.

As we talked, it became obvious she was using chocolate to control her stress. She's not the only person doing that. Nowadays it is common to use something external to change how we feel – whether we are stressed, overwhelmed or just bored. Drinking, drugs, sex, alcohol, television and burying yourself in work are common ways of changing how we feel, but the world's favourite by far is sugar.

The actress was controlling her stress, but she felt she was not able to have just one piece of chocolate. She had to demolish the whole bar. In other words, the chocolate was in charge, not her.

I showed her a safer way to deal with stress, and using the following technique we completely changed her relationship to chocolate. It only took a few minutes. Afterwards she could look at bar of chocolate and be free to eat one piece or none at all. She could take it or leave it.

Twenty-one seconds

I hear people saying things like, 'It takes twenty-one days to change a habit.' But I have seen people change a lifetime habit in just twenty-one seconds. People can reorient their feelings and make life-changing decisions in a single moment.

My techniques often involve creating visualizations and intense emotional feelings and then attaching them to new ways of thinking and behaving. Don't be too surprised at how the Craving Buster helps you to feel more in control about food, particularly sugar.

Let me explain why the Craving Buster works so well. It uses conditioning and the power of the imagination. One hundred years ago physiologist Ivan Pavlov discovered the power of conditioning when he induced salivation in dogs just by ringing a bell. He created this reaction by ringing a bell every time he was about to feed his dogs. The dogs soon learned to associate the sound of the bell with the arrival of food so they began salivating as soon as they heard the bell. Pavlov had conditioned his dogs to respond to the bell. We can use the same principle to create a conditioned response that will change your response to a sugary food or drink.

We use the power of the imagination because the imagination is more powerful than the will. For example, you can't speed up your heart by willpower alone. However, if you vividly imagine being in a dangerous or frightening place, such as hearing footsteps behind you in a dark alley at night or being chased by an angry mob, your heart will speed up.

We use these two psychological techniques to program your brain to link a compulsion with a repulsion. One cancels out the other so that next time you see that drink or food you will be able to take it or leave it.

I would like you now to think of a sugary food or beverage that you crave and are out of control around. It could be chocolate or anything else that is a sugar problem for you.

Now we are going to get your brain to re-create the feeling of compulsion for the food or beverage you crave and blend it with your physical reaction to food that revolts you. When the compulsion food simultaneously triggers repulsion, one feeling will cancel out the other. Then you are free to choose whether you want to eat or drink or not.

I have to tell you that this technique will be uncomfortable for a few moments, because you need to get a very strong feeling of revulsion to cancel out the compulsion, but don't worry. The discomfort is well worth it!

THE CRAVING BUSTER

Read through every step of this technique before you do it. If you want me to help you, put the CD on and I will walk you through it one step at a time.

Before we start, I'd like you to rate your craving for the sugary food that you feel out of control around on a scale of 1–10, with 1 being the lowest and 10 the highest. This is important, because in a moment we want to know how much it's reduced. Make a note now of where the craving is on that scale.

1. Think of a food that absolutely revolts you, so that even if you just think of it you feel slightly nauseous. This is stronger than dislike. I need you to feel seriously uncomfortable in order to restore your power. When I ask people to think of a food that makes them feel sick, they say everything from chopped liver to broccoli. Imagine a plate of whatever you really hate in front of you now.

2. Now, as vividly as possible, imagine eating that food now. Taste it, feel the texture in your mouth and the awful feeling of swallowing it, again and again.

3. Keep doing it again and again until you feel really revolted.

4. Now imagine adding some of the sugary food or drink that you feel out of control around to the food you feel revolted by. Mix the taste and texture as you chew and taste them together. It feels disgusting.

5. Now imagine adding the hair from the floor of a hairdresser's to the food mixture. Taste how they all feel together and experience the texture in your mouth with all those hairs, and really chew them before you try to swallow them.

6. Now, continuing to experience the taste and texture of the food that makes you feel sick, mixed with the food you used to like, mixed with hairs, and add the taste of a bucket of spit and let all the tastes mix together in your mouth until you feel utterly revolted.

7. Next vividly imagine swallowing them together. It must taste disgusting!

8. Now, think about the food you felt out of control of and rate your desire on a scale of 1–10. It should be significantly lower now. If you want to make it lower still, go over the steps again to make yourself feel even more revolted before you add the food you liked.

9. When you can think about the food you were out of control around and can take it or leave it, you are back in control.

IN A NUTSHELL

- Sugar is a deadly, slow-motion killer

- Reducing your sugar intake will massively improve your health

- Use the mind-programming process every day for the next seven days

- Use the journal every day to track your success

- Use the Craving Buster to switch off desire for problem food or drink

2

·

THE GREAT SUGAR CONSPIRACY

THE GREAT SUGAR CONSPIRACY

Perhaps you are now thinking what I did when I started this project. I asked myself:

If sugar is really this bad . . .
and if the science is so clear . . .
and if the research has been going on since the 1960s . . .
why haven't I heard all this before?

More importantly, why is sugar consumption still increasing when the damage it causes is manifest all around us? The answer is devastating. Science and medicine have been subverted by big business. Money triumphed over health. People are dying all over the world while corporate fat cats get rich.

It starts with a man called Ancel Keys

In the 1950s an American physiologist named Ancel Keys developed a theory that eating fat caused heart attacks. Keys published the 'Seven Countries' study which appeared to show that the more fat people ate, the higher their blood cholesterol levels. He believed high cholesterol led to heart disease.

Ancel Keys' study started out as a 22-country study but, for some unknown reason, in the end he used data from only seven countries. That produced a nice neat graph apparently showing an exact correlation between fat consumption and cholesterol.

It is strange, however, that he omitted France, Switzerland and West Germany, which had low rates of heart disease and diets high in fat. If the data available from all twenty-two countries is included, the correlation looks like nonsense.

Keys left out data from Crete, where almost 40 per cent of the diet is fat yet the heart-disease deaths were the lowest in the study. The study also ignored data from the Masai (in Africa) who live exclusively on meat and dairy, and Inuit (in North America) who lived on fish and meat for nine months of the year, and yet had the lowest rates of heart disease on the planet.

Professor George Mann of Vanderbilt University, who had studied the Masai, described the notion that fat is the cause of heart disease as 'the greatest scam in the history of medicine'. Unfortunately, people did not pay attention to Dr Mann. They were listening to Keys.

Professor John Yudkin

While Keys was working in the USA, Professor John Yudkin established the department of nutrition at Queen Elizabeth College, London. Yudkin distrusted Keys' work and conducted his own research into sugar. Throughout the 1960s he conducted experiments and investigations which demonstrated over and over again the dangers of sugar.

While I was researching this book, I was surprised to find out that my mother knew Professor Yudkin. At that time she was a lecturer training teachers of home economics in Enfield. Her students were expected to attend one of Dr Yudkin's lectures every term so she met him many times and had a friendly professional relationship with him. She and all her colleagues admired him and were disgusted at how he was treated by the establishment.

Yudkin was mild-mannered and was always both correct and gentlemanly in presenting his findings. Keys was not, and he attacked both Yudkin and his findings, calling one of Yudkin's papers 'a mountain of nonsense'.

The attack by the sugar industry

In 1972 Yudkin published *Pure, White and Deadly*, a summary of his research to date and a powerful warning of the dangers of sugar. The sugar industry immediately tried to discredit him. The World Sugar Research Organisation called his book 'science fiction'. The British Sugar Bureau dismissed his book as 'emotional assertions', although the book could not have been more careful, measured and scientific. Yudkin was persistently attacked by sugar industry bodies and their allies in academia. He found that invitations to conferences were withdrawn, and on several occasions when he did present papers at conferences they were not published in the subsequent literature.

The British Nutrition Foundation (BNF) was set up in 1967, funded by the food industry. Very soon it was pressuring Yudkin to stop talking about sugar. The large food companies that sponsored the BNF threatened to withdraw their support if Yudkin was appointed to the body, although he was by far the most appropriate person. Throughout the 1960s and 1970s the sugar industry and their stooges continued to attack Yudkin and his theories. Every attempt Yudkin made at constructive discussion was rebuffed or undermined.

Sugar and tobacco

In 1965 the Sugar Research Foundation, backed by the US sugar industry, paid scientists to conduct a literature review published in the prestigious *New England Journal of Medicine*. It focused on fat as the cause of cardiovascular disease and minimized sugar. This one document misrepresented a whole field of research. It was an unforgiveable distortion of science, minimizing health risks to boost corporate profit.

We know about the involvement of the Sugar Research Foundation because of investigations by Cristin Kearns and Stanton Glantz published in 2016. Stanton Glantz is the academic who unearthed the evidence that the tobacco industry deliberately concealed the dangers of tobacco for decades.

Sugar and tobacco have too much in common.

From the 1950s to the 1980s the US food industry had a good friend in Dr Frederick Stare, the head of the department of nutrition at Harvard. Over his career, Stare obtained many millions of dollars of funding from major food and beverage companies for the Harvard School of Public Health and the Nutrition Foundation. He steadfastly defended sugar and in 1975 edited a laughable compilation of pro-sugar arguments that were to be used prolifically by the sugar industry.

A shameful campaign

The campaign against Yudkin and his ideas was long, sustained and disgraceful, but for twenty-five years it was successful. Doctors, researchers and nutritionists more or less ignored sugar. They all focused on reducing fat in diets, and alarmingly many professionals to this day consider that eating fat is the main factor in heart disease and obesity. They are wrong.

A large-scale controlled study in 1993 showed that a low-fat diet had no benefit whatsoever in reducing incidence of heart disease. A Europe-wide study in 2008 showed results directly opposed to the 'fat makes you sick' hypothesis. France had the highest intake of saturated fat and the lowest rate of heart disease; Ukraine had the lowest intake of saturated fat and the highest rate of heart disease. A United Nations review in the same year found no link between fat, heart disease and cancer. The science clearly shows that fat is not significant.

The tragedy of Ancel Keys' legacy is not just that he was wrong, but that his ideas have made things worse. His hypothesis became almost universally accepted. It underpinned the official US government advice to limit intake of dietary fat. In many foods fat has been replaced by sugar. From 1971 to 2006 the percentage of calories from fat in the average American's diet fell by 3 per cent. During that time obesity doubled and rates of heart disease and diabetes continued relentlessly upwards, year after year.

The truth about fat

In 2000 a journalist called Nina Teicholz started working as a restaurant reviewer. For the first time in her life she was regularly eating rich, fatty, meaty meals. To her astonishment she lost more and more weight. She was so bewildered that she set out to research the established view that fat makes people fat. She came across Ancel Keys' study and she soon found the flaws in it. She also found the scientists who disagreed with Keys. Teicholz spent over a decade meticulously researching the whole area and eventually published her findings in a book called *The Big Fat Surprise: Why Butter, Meat and Cheese Belong in a Healthy Diet*.

The book became a *New York Times* bestseller, but Teicholz came under repeated attack by professionals in the field of nutrition. There are scientists who still cling to the Keys hypothesis, despite all the evidence that has accrued to show it is false. It always seems to me that when someone is attacked personally, the attackers have run out of legitimate arguments. Like Professor Yudkin, Teicholz has been attacked for speaking an inconvenient truth.

Low-fat, high-sugar

Ancel Keys' advice was a huge market opportunity for the food industry. From the 1960s onwards the industry was expanding massively, selling ready-made 'convenience' foods. Now, using industrial processes, they could remove fat from everyday foods and market their new products as healthy 'low-fat' options. Of course, they continued to sell high-fat versions as well to cover the whole market.

Unfortunately 'low-fat' often means bad taste or no taste at all. Much of the taste of food is carried in the fat. To make up for the lack of taste caused by removing fat, the industry added sugar.

Now their products were not only useless in terms of disease prevention, they were actively damaging. Low-fat became high-sugar. And high-sugar is far, far worse than fat. High-sugar causes the very heart disease low-fat was sold to prevent.

The money-making machine

The world had changed and millions of people were to die over the next thirty years as the food manufacturers got rich. The conditions were perfect for the expansion of diet clubs. Sugar was causing people to get fatter but the truth was being hidden. The clubs sold manufactured low-fat artificial foods that were worse than useless; they were able to keep their members trapped, forever trying to lose weight and forever failing.

Diet clubs and supermarkets still sell low-fat products loaded up with sugar, and many advisory bodies and health charities still tell people to eat low-fat and make no mention of sugar.

It may be no coincidence that many such advisory bodies have advisors with strong links to the food industry. In 2015 the *BMJ* (British Medical Journal) published a remarkable diagram laying bare the network of relationships between key public health experts and vast sums of money provided by the food industry.

Food and drink manufacturers are in business to make money. They do not have a duty to protect public health. They make money by producing what people buy, and people still buy vast quantities of sugary drinks and food with added sugar.

Food is very big business. Just ten companies are behind the brands which make up 90 per cent of all the food in the average supermarket.

Food manufacturers can point out that sugar is not only a taste that people like. It is also a very useful ingredient if you want to manufacture food in bulk and keep it palatable for days, weeks or months before it reaches the consumer. It is a traditional ingredient in many dishes. It is a flavour enhancer and a flavour disguiser. It is used to enhance mouthfeel and to help food stay fresh longer. It is used as a preservative. And of course if it is only consumed occasionally, it is not dangerous.

But they know sugar is dangerous

Prize-winning reporter Michael Moss uncovered evidence of a meeting in 1999 of the chief executives of the biggest food manufacturers in the United States. They heard a presentation which made an explicit link between the industry and the problem of obesity in the United States. It proposed steps to address the problem. These steps included reducing the amounts of sugar, salt and fat in processed foods and embracing a code to limit advertising to children.

The proposals were rejected. One chief executive stated bluntly that he was providing what the consumer wanted to buy. His company produced foods containing sugar and fat. As long as the consumers were buying, his company would continue to sell.

Big businesses don't just make a product and then hope people like it. They spend enormous sums of money developing and researching their products. They engineer their food to hit the exact spot where the combination of tastes is as delicious as possible before it becomes overwhelming. Psychologist Howard Moskowitz called it the 'bliss point'. He built his very successful career with a system of collating and analysing feedback from consumers to build the perfect version of each product. Moskowitz worked on everything from spaghetti sauce to soft drinks and his work has helped to sell billions of dollars' worth of product.

Cravings by design

The most delicious taste possible sounds brilliant. It should be making us all deliriously happy, shouldn't it? Perfect food! But that is not the ultimate goal of big food companies. They don't want to sell you the perfect food. They want to sell you the food that is most likely to make you want to buy more.

That is why so many processed foods are absolutely delicious when you put them in your mouth but leave you strangely unsatisfied afterwards. That is not an accident. It is deliberate. If a food product had a delicious aftertaste that lingered like a fine wine, people would eat it more slowly. They would eat less of it. They would enjoy that aftertaste and notice more swiftly the signals of satiety from their stomach.

Technologists in food product design laboratories make sure that the pleasurable part of the taste finishes swiftly but there is enough sugar or salt to keep you salivating and wanting more. They spend huge sums of money creating these foods. Snack manufacturers even have machines to measure the crunchiness of crisps to find the perfect breaking point. There is nothing accidental about snacks that make you eat too much and leave you unsatisfied.

When you find you ate more crisps or sweets or pizza than you intended, you probably blamed yourself for being greedy. Stop blaming yourself. If you want to blame anyone, try blaming the manufacturer who undermined your satiety system to keep you eating.

More sugar, more sales

The trio of ingredients that make people want to eat more are sugar, fat and salt, and the worst of the three, by a long, long, long way, is sugar. As we shall see it is also the most effective at creating a desire for more food, and specifically for more sugar.

Sugar is added to 75 per cent of the products in your local supermarket. The more products with added sugar people buy, the more they are likely to buy in the future. No wonder manufacturers like to add sugar to their products. It does their marketing for them.

Advertising

It is sickening that so many dangerous, sugar-laden foods are sold as 'part of a healthy diet' and millions upon millions of pounds have been spent on associating sugar-filled drinks with health, love and friendship. So much money is spent advertising food that no politician and none of the mainstream media can afford to ban it or challenge it. We have to defend ourselves. These three rules of thumb are my personal defences against advertising:

1. **The more a food is advertised, the more sugar it is likely to contain.**

This appears to be true nine times out of ten. It is probably because only the really big companies can afford big advertising budgets and the big companies make highly processed food. Sugar is a key ingredient of processed food.

2. **If it is aimed at children, there is almost certainly sugar in it.**

Children can be fussy eaters but are easily seduced by sugar. Manufacturers know this and add sugar to almost everything aimed at children – even baby food!

3. The picture always lies: beautiful, thin people don't eat garbage.

Whenever you see a beautiful model eating or drinking a processed food product, you can pretty much guarantee they would never touch it in real life. People don't look that good by eating junk.

Defence against advertising

Perhaps the most famous television advert of all time was made in 1971 to advertise a soft drink. A group of young people from all over the world were gathered on a hillside to lip-sync a super-catchy jingle about peace, love and a soft drink. The jingle was so popular it was soon made into a pop song. I realized as I looked at the ad on YouTube that if you were to assemble the same number of young Americans on a hillside now you would need a bigger hillside. Only a third of them would be a healthy weight. One third would be overweight, and the last third would be obese.

If you are old enough to remember that advert, visualize it like that now: a group of fat people singing. Remember, it is not even their fault they are fat. Soft drink companies don't print any warnings on their bottles or cans, and every person who drinks a can of soda every day is damaging their own satiety signalling. They aren't getting the signal, 'You need to stop.'

This advert was the inspiration for my technique for defending myself against sugary advertising.

DEFENCE AGAINST ADVERTISING

Read it through first, then practise applying it to an advert you can remember. Run through it as many times as you need so that when you next see an advert for a drink or food that is heavy in sugar, you can use it immediately.

1. Bring to mind an advertisement for a soft drink, fast-food brand or branded food product that contains sugar.
2. Note how many people appear in it, both adults and children, including all cartoon characters.
3. Now rerun the advertisement in your mind recasting every character, including cartoon characters, with an obese adult or child you have recently seen.

IN A NUTSHELL

- Natural fats are perfectly healthy

- Low-fat leads to high-sugar

- Good scientists have known for over forty years that sugar is dangerous

- Junk food is designed to make you crave more

- Edit every advert for processed foods to feature fat people

3

·

THE SCIENCE
OF SUGAR
MADE EASY

THE SCIENCE OF SUGAR MADE EASY

Now let's look at the facts. By the time you have finished this chapter, you will understand why sugar is so dangerous and you will be started on the path to freedom.

I have carefully picked out here the essential science you need to know. If you want to know a bit more you can read the tint sections on pages 65, 78–9 and 83, but if science is not your thing it is not necessary to do so. If you are really interested, there is a further reading list at the end of the journal. All you need to do now is read the main text so that you and your unconscious mind know all you need to know to make the changes that will free you from sugar.

Please do read this section. It is short and even if you do not understand immediately, relax and your unconscious mind will act on the suggestions I make during the mind-programming relaxation. Just read it through and don't worry if you don't completely understand it straight away. By the time you have finished the book, you will understand more about sugar than 99 per cent of the population.

How we digest our food

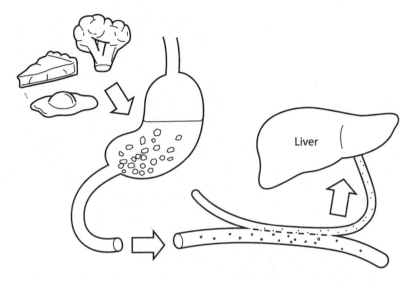

Our bodies extract energy from food without any help from the conscious mind. The whole process is automatic, run by the autonomic nervous system and neuropeptide networks, so when you eat, your food is broken down in your stomach and gut and the nutrients pass through the walls of your intestine into your bloodstream. Foods such as bread, beans, vegetables, potatoes and pasta all contain carbohydrates, which are broken down into glucose as they enter your bloodstream. A hormone called insulin helps the body take in the glucose where it is needed. Fats and protein are broken down into amino acids and fatty acids and used to repair the cells of your body, provide energy or be stored as fat.

Blood sugar

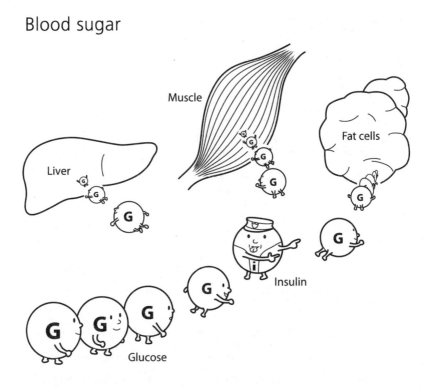

Glucose is your fuel. You need glucose all the time in your bloodstream, where it is known as 'blood sugar'. The cells in your body use it to stay alive. Your level of blood sugar needs to stay within a certain range. Too little and you die swiftly, too much and you die very slowly.

When your blood sugar rises above a certain level, your pancreas releases insulin. Insulin is your body's traffic controller. It opens the cell walls to allow the muscles, liver and fat cells to take in the glucose and store it for later usage. In your muscles and liver, the glucose molecules are stuck together and stored as glycogen, which is a quick-release energy store. If the muscles and liver have enough glucose, the rest is converted to fat and stored in fat cells.

As blood sugar is used up, the liver releases glucose back into the bloodstream to maintain a healthy level.

Your liver is like a battery, charging up when you eat, then slowly discharging to keep you going between meals.

Burning glucose

All the cells in your body use glucose. They contain little power stations that break down glucose in a series of chemical reactions to release energy. This series of chemical reactions has a feedback loop so that when there is enough energy in the cell, the process stops. When more energy is required, it restarts.

The simple overview

Your body detects what you are eating and produces the necessary enzymes and hormones to break it down and deliver the nutrients where they are needed. Glucose is stored in the cells, and when energy is needed it is broken down, releasing energy.

So why is sugar deadly?

Everything I said above is true for all food *except* sugar. Let's have a closer look at sugar now. The scientific name for everyday sugar is 'sucrose'. There are some other carbohydrates which scientists call 'sugars' (see the box opposite) but when I refer to sugar in this text, I am referring to sucrose.

Sucrose is made of two other molecules, glucose and fructose, stuck together. Fructose is the bad part.

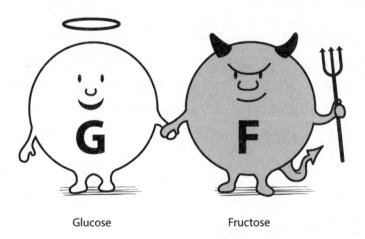

Glucose   Fructose

THE DIFFERENT SUGARS

There are several different molecules called 'sugars' by scientists. They are all carbohydrates, made of carbon, hydrogen and oxygen.

- The simple sugars (called 'monosaccharides') are glucose, fructose and galactose.
- The compound sugars ('disaccharides'), made of two monosaccharides stuck together, are lactose, maltose and sucrose.
- The everyday substance we call 'sugar' is sucrose.
- In the digestive process all the sugars, with the exception of fructose, are eventually broken down to glucose.
- In the USA, manufacturers use a lot of high-fructose corn syrup (HFCS). Some people worry that it is worse than ordinary sugar (sucrose). It is not. It has just the same effect on the body. High-fructose corn syrup and sucrose are both sweet, they both break down to fructose and glucose in the body, and they both cause exactly the same damage.

Why is fructose so deadly?

The liver is the only organ that can use fructose. The process to break down fructose inside the liver has no feedback loop. As long as there is fructose, the process will carry on. When it produces more energy than the liver can handle, the liver turns the excess into fatty acids. Some are stored in the liver as fat, which damages your liver, some are pumped out into the bloodstream and some end up in fat cells. Now the liver, and your bloodstream, have too much fat. If all that seems too complicated remember this:

Your body turns sugar into fat.

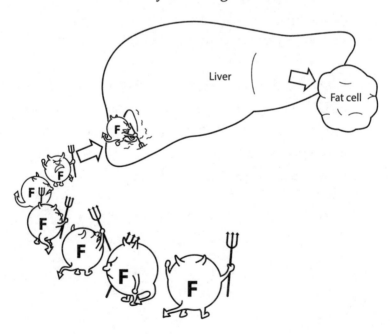

How sugar causes heart disease

Sugar raises levels of fatty acids and cholesterol in your bloodstream. There has been a lot of confusion and bad advice about cholesterol over the years. Cholesterol, it turns out, is mostly good for you. Even what used to be called 'bad' cholesterol is mostly harmless. However, there is just one type of so-called 'bad' cholesterol, called 'small dense low-density lipoproteins,' or 'small dense LDL' for short, which really is bad. And that is the type that fructose tends to create.

Small dense LDL sticks to the walls of arteries and clogs them up. That makes the heart work harder and raises blood pressure. Sometimes a big lump of it can build up and then break off into the bloodstream and cause a stroke or a heart attack. The bottom line is:

**Sugar massively increases the risk of
strokes and heart attacks.**

The big breakfast disaster

That's enough science for now. We don't have to know the whole story before we start to change things for the better. Let's begin at the beginning of the day.

The modern British breakfast is a disaster. Millions of people start every day with a glass of juice and a bowl of cereal. The old joke was that there was more nutrition in the box than in the cereal. It still has the ring of truth.

Almost all cereals are upwards of 20 per cent sugar. There are one or two which are as low as 10 per cent, but most of them are more than one-fifth pure sugar by weight.

Many adverts emphasize the fruit or fibre or vitamin or mineral content, but that content is an unimportant distraction. The quantities required and delivered are both tiny and you will get all the fibre, vitamins and minerals you need from a few vegetables later in the day.

The elephant in the breakfast bowl is sugar. People who start the day with sugar are more likely to want more sugar during the day. The craving is both habitual and physical.

On the other hand, the old-fashioned breakfast of bacon and eggs is a far healthier start to the day. But just before you decide

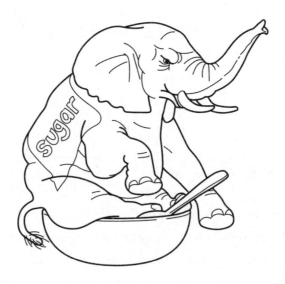

you have to eat bacon and eggs every morning for the rest of your life, let me tell you about other breakfasts. In Northern Europe people often start the day with ham or cheese. In most parts of Asia breakfast is a meal which looks just like lunch or dinner. It could be rice or noodles or meat or fish.

And of course there are just a few cereals that contain no sugar at all. If you want to find them, read the labels very, very carefully.

A better way to start your day

People eat cereals because they are quick and convenient and because they have been relentlessly advertised for decades. Many people have been so powerfully influenced that they find it difficult to imagine breakfast without cereal.

I want you to have a far better start to your day. So I'm going to ask you to do two things: make one change one day this week, and use a powerful psychological technique to embed a new direction in your unconscious mind.

One change per week makes all the difference

If you have usually been eating a sugary cereal for breakfast, then one day this week, change your breakfast to exclude sugar. Don't change everything all at once, just try this for one day. Of course if you notice how much better you feel straight away, feel free to carry on. But if you are not sure, or you need more assistance to change your habits, change your breakfast on just one day this week and make a note in your journal.

Next week have a sugar-free breakfast on two days. The following week, three days, and so on, until by the time you reach the end of your journal you are heading for six sugar-free breakfasts a week.

Program your mind for a healthy future

We must reprogram your unconscious mind to move towards a healthy future. We will have a look at a negative version of reality, so that we can steer your mind towards a positive future. We will give your unconscious mind something to move away from and something to move towards.

This technique sets up the unconscious mind to help steer you away from sources of sugar that you do not normally think about. As your awareness grows of how much sugar is in the food environment, your knowledge will be integrated and you will find that there is a real pull towards feeling healthy every day and letting that feeling guide you more and more powerfully to a healthy future.

PROGRAM YOUR MIND FOR A HEALTHY FUTURE

Read this exercise through from beginning to end before you start to do it. Then take four or five minutes to go through it, vividly imagining each step. Most people prefer to do this with me, so please use the CD and let me guide you.

Do this exercise at least once, more often if you like. Once you have vividly shown it to your unconscious mind, the positive direction will be set and we will reinforce it every time you listen to the mind-programming.

You need to be somewhere you can safely close your eyes for ten minutes and remain undisturbed.

Often people find they are a little uncomfortable doing this exercise. If at any point you feel you are becoming too upset, stop using it because it is not for you.

Now we are going to imagine two completely different futures.

1. Relax and close your eyes and imagine you are near the end of your life. In this vision you have continued through life eating sugar recklessly, and knowing what you know now about the dangers of sugar, let your unconscious mind begin to show you what your health could be like . . . It could be in old age that you suffered from diabetes or heart disease or cancer. Did you have a stroke, or a heart attack? You may see a vision of yourself in a hospital bed or very ill, with the people you love around you looking sad.

2. In this vision, what would this older, sicker self say to the younger you to make you value and protect your health and family?

3. Let your unconscious review this vision and, when it has taken the messages it needs to lead you to health, the vision will fade.

4. Now imagine a second vision in which you are near the end of a wonderful life, in which you used this book to seriously and permanently reduce your sugar intake. You are older but healthy. You are grateful for long years of health and happiness, surrounded by your friends and family. From this perspective of a healthy old age, what advice would this wise older person give you right now?

5. Let your unconscious review this vision and, when it has taken the messages it needs to lead you to health, the vision will fade.

6. Now create a still, black and white picture of the vision of ill-health from excess sugar and imagine it to your left.

7. Now imagine a bigger, colourful, brighter picture of your healthy, happy old age and place it to your right.

8. Imagine them both, and now make the picture of sickness smaller and move it so it is three times further away. At the same time, make the picture of health bigger, brighter, bolder and closer.

9. Whenever you need a conscious boost of healthiness and motivation, repeat steps 6, 7 and 8.

IN A NUTSHELL

- Your body turns fructose into fat

- Fructose is bad for your heart and your arteries

- Start your day without sugar

- Visualize your happy, healthy, sugar-free future

4

·

SUGAR AND FEELING FULL

SUGAR AND FEELING FULL

We have seen some of the damage sugar does, but the reason sugar is such a big problem is that it disrupts the balance of your body's natural control system.

The science behind this is very important but we don't need to know about every detail. All the key points are in the main text. If you find science fascinating and want to explore it in detail, see the tint sections on pages 65, 78–9 and 83 and go to the further reading list at the end, after the journal.

You don't need to be an electrician to switch on a light and you don't need to be a mechanic to drive a car. In the same way, you don't have to study medicine or psychology to change your behaviour.

Read the main text at least once. Your unconscious mind will soak it in and use it to make changes while you are listening to the mind-programming.

How do you know when you have had enough to eat?

That sounds like a funny question, because we hardly ever ask it. We just feel full and stop eating. We don't find the answer by a lot of thinking. The feeling of fullness has a special name: satiety.

Your brain continuously monitors the process of digestion. Every one of the hormones involved in digesting your food is involved in signalling to your brain that you are full. So as you eat, you feel full. It is a very efficient system. For more details, see the box overleaf. The important point is this:

**The hormones released during digestion
tell your brain when you are full.**

THE HORMONES OF SATIETY

Food is vital for our survival, so the body has multiple overlapping systems that monitor and control our energy supply. The hormones that control the digestion of food continually signal our state and our requirements to the brain. Some create hunger to push us to eat, and others reward us with satiety. Insulin, CCK and leptin are the main hormones driving satiety, but other hormones affect your appetite too.

Ghrelin

When your stomach is empty, ghrelin is released. Your hypothalamus, a part of your brain, reacts to the ghrelin and makes you hungry. When you eat, ghrelin levels reduce and you feel less hungry.

Insulin

When you eat, glucose rises in your bloodstream so your pancreas starts to produce insulin. Insulin helps to store the glucose. When the insulin reaches a certain level in the bloodstream, the hypothalamus responds to it and triggers the feeling of satiety.

Cholecystokinin (CKK)

Cholecystokinin is released when you eat fat and proteins. CCK also signals the hypothalamus to trigger satiety. It switches off hunger when you have eaten enough to meet the body's requirements.

Leptin

When you finish eating, insulin and CCK are no longer needed, so their levels fall quite rapidly. That would make you feel unsatisfied quite quickly too, and hungry again, but if in fact you do have enough energy on board, it is stored in your fat cells so they release another hormone called leptin. Leptin tells the hypothalamus that you still have plenty of energy and you don't yet need to eat.

GLP1 & PYY

GLP1 both stimulates the production of insulin and signals satiety. PYY is released later in the digestion process and inhibits insulin secretion and helps the colon reabsorb water and electrolytes. It also signals satiety.

How sugar screws it all up

The natural system of satiety or fullness signalling is very elegant and it worked wonderfully for almost everyone for tens of thousands of years until about forty years ago. It started to go seriously wrong when people started to eat serious amounts of sugar. Sugar, specifically the fructose part, makes a complete mess of your satiety system.

When your liver processes fructose it doesn't trigger any of the hormones that signal satiety. So it never makes your brain feel that you are full.

Fructose doesn't trigger the feeling of fullness.

The big insight

When I found out that sugar fails to trigger the feeling of fullness, it made sense of something that had bothered me for years. Whenever I ate fast food or sweets or biscuits or ready meals, I noticed that I enjoyed them at the time, but somehow I never felt really satisfied. I could even feel physically full because my stomach was tight, but I never seemed to reach contentment. It was as though my feelings of 'full up' or 'hungry' got blurred. I was never starving, but I always believed I wanted a bit more. Now I had the explanation.

Doesn't the glucose bit help?

If you've been following the science closely you'll realize that there seems to be a possible solution. Remember sucrose, everyday sugar, is made of two molecules: fructose and glucose. We have found out that fructose is a problem, but surely the glucose part should still trigger satiety? We know that a rise in glucose levels makes your pancreas release insulin and that should still trigger satiety, even if it takes a bit longer to do so.

The worst that could happen *should* be that we eat twice as much sugar as we need and then feel full because of the effect of the glucose. We *should* be OK.

And that is indeed what happens, provided that you are not a regular or chronic sugar-eater. If you eat very small amounts of sugar your liver won't get overwhelmed and the system will still work.

If you only eat sugar-rich foods like cake or desserts once a week, you are likely to eat a bit more than usual, but you will feel full and very soon your body's system is re-established and works as well as ever.

Unfortunately, that is not what happens to people who consume more than very small amounts of sugar on a daily basis. The vast majority of people eat too much sugar and they drink too much sugar.

The dark danger of chronic sugar consumption

Chronic fructose consumption makes the liver fatty and that causes 'insulin resistance', a condition in which insulin stops working properly. The pancreas therefore has to make more insulin. When there is a lot of insulin and a lot of glucose in the bloodstream, the brain stops recognizing the 'fullness' signals. The knock-on effect disables all the other 'fullness' hormones too.

Regular sugar consumption switches off all your body's hormonal fullness signals.

Luckily, even this dangerous situation can be reversed. However, it is vital that you use all the techniques in this book as directed. When you do so, your body will respond correctly to those signals again, and you will be guided back to your natural state of balance and health.

INSULIN RESISTANCE AND THE DESTRUCTION OF SATIETY

1. Fructose is turned to fatty acids in your bloodstream, which get stored as fat in the liver and around the organs in the middle of your body.

2. Fat in the liver has a name: Non Alcoholic Fatty Liver Disease or NAFLD for short. NAFLD damages your liver.

3. Fatty acids in the bloodstream and NAFLD cause insulin resistance, the condition in which insulin doesn't work properly.

4. Insulin resistance is progressive, which means that if food intake remains the same, the condition gets worse and worse. The pancreas has to produce more and more insulin just to get the glucose into your muscles and liver.

5. Insulin resistance switches off satiety. Insulin no longer tells the brain you are full. Insulin also inhibits the effect of leptin. Soon there are no hormones at all telling the brain to stop eating.

6. Satiety is switched off temporarily by a surge of fructose, but with insulin resistance it becomes chronically dysfunctional. As long as there is insulin resistance, satiety is at best impaired and at worst disabled.

7. When satiety is disabled, a person has no hormonal signalling of fullness regardless of whatever food they are eating. Chronic sugar-eaters eat too much of anything they eat.

Sick, fat and still eating

Sugar-eaters end up with high blood sugar, high insulin and high levels of fatty acids in the bloodstream, but they are not getting the signals to stop eating. This is the reason that sugar is such a global disaster. Sugar makes people sick and fat, and it disables the control system that should save them. It should not be possible for so many people to be so overweight and yet keep overeating. But sugar has dismantled their defences.

The last defence

As well as the hormones I have mentioned, there is one more pathway to the brain that tells us we are full. The final signal of satiety comes from the stomach. When the stomach is full, nerve endings in the stomach wall sense it is being stretched and signal to the brain to stop eating. The trouble, however, is that if someone is eating too much sugar and has already enlarged their stomach, this signal is arriving too late, and they keep stretching their stomachs and making them bigger and bigger. This explains why some sugar-eaters were telling me that *even when their stomach hurt* they didn't really feel full.

Sugar works like a virus on a computer. Once it gets behind the defences it disables them from the inside, so there is no longer a hormonal limit to the amount of sugar or any other food that people can take in. The system in this book will erase that virus.

Sugar causes obesity

Years ago I had a hunch that sugar was not healthy because so many people told me that some form of sugar was their weak point. For some it was colas and soft drinks, for others it was the secret biscuit stash in the desk at their office. However, I believed then, as I do now, that everyone is capable of being guided to eat well by their own appetite.

Another reason I looked at sugar again was because of the success of my book *I Can Make You Thin*. Follow-up research showed that the system is successful for seven out of ten people, which is far more successful than any diet or any other weight-loss method. But I wanted to know why it was not ten out of ten.

I found out that some people lacked motivation and others did not follow the instructions properly, but I also found some people who genuinely found it very, very difficult to sense when they had had enough to eat. I now understand that those people were struggling because sugar had seriously impaired or switched off their satiety.

Sugar is no ordinary food. Sugar messes with the body's control system and that is why those people were having so much trouble. When chronic sugar consumption has set up insulin resistance, people can eat too much sugar and too much of anything else and still fail to feel properly satisfied.

Feeling full and hunger

So right now, we must start to restore your ability to feel full and completely satisfied. For each person, this will take a different amount of time, depending on how much sugar you have been consuming. As you reduce your intake of sugar, insulin resistance will reduce naturally, but regardless of how much or how little sugar you have consumed, you can start to restore your satiety right now.

Along with restored satiety, you will restore your authentic, natural hunger too. When satiety is damaged, hunger is damaged too. Sugar-eaters never feel properly full and never feel properly hungry. They always have a nagging sense they would like a bit more, but they never feel as though they are really, properly, physically hungry.

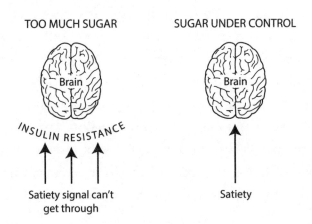

TOO MUCH SUGAR   SUGAR UNDER CONTROL

Brain   Brain

INSULIN RESISTANCE

Satiety signal can't get through   Satiety

You will discover that along with really feeling satisfied by a good meal, you will also experience proper, motivating hunger, which builds up naturally and gradually before you eat.

RESET YOUR FULLNESS SIGNAL

1. Cut out snacks. Don't worry – you will be able to eat them again just as soon as you have restored your natural control system. The chances are you will eat fewer in the future anyway, but right now, while you recalibrate, we need you to stop eating snacks. First, this will of course reduce sugar intake, because so many snacks contain sugar. Secondly, it will allow your hunger to build naturally and slowly between meals.

2. Help yourself to good portions when you eat your meals, but wait for twenty minutes if you wish to have seconds. While your satiety is impaired it can take up to twenty minutes for your stomach and your brain to register whether you really need any more food.

3. Ensure that you are taking at least a moderate amount of exercise five days a week. You don't have to join a gym or run a marathon. Just thirty minutes of walking or other exercise will reduce insulin resistance and hence restore satiety.

4. Listen to the mind-programming process on the CD every day for seven days. There are special suggestions during the relaxation section that will boost your normal satiety system.

It is not your fault

When satiety goes wrong, we feel something is wrong but it is difficult to put our finger on it. Some people know they are emotional eaters; others don't really understand, they just feel uncomfortable. It is a relief to find out that when sugar has damaged your control system, it is not your fault it's not working.

Now you know how to fix it. As you use this system, you will reduce sugar at your own speed and you will find that your natural appetite and your natural satiety will return. This process will work regardless of the speed at which you change, so remember that although you didn't cause the problem, you now have the solution.

Visualization

The next technique makes use of your brain's ability to visualize. Occasionally I meet people who tell me they can't visualize. It often turns out that they think I am asking them to hallucinate! Visualization is a simple process that we all use, often without paying much attention. Let me show you. Please answer this question: 'On which side of your front door is the lock?' In order to answer, you created a mental picture of your door. That is visualization, and that is all you need.

Swish

This technique was developed by my good friend and colleague Dr Richard Bandler, who has devoted his life to harnessing the practical power of the mind. Richard found that people use internal pictures with emotional significance to guide their decisions.

For example, imagine you have been invited to a party. If the image that springs to mind is one of people smiling and laughing, having a good time and enjoying each other's company, you will probably feel like going to the party. If, on the other hand, the picture is one of individuals standing around looking awkward, or a few loud, boring people getting drunk, you are unlikely to want to go to the party.

We automatically make pictures like this while we make decisions, and the process can happen so fast we hardly notice we are doing it.

In order to make new, better decisions, we are going to redirect your imagery deliberately over and over again until it creates new automatic preferences which will replace ones that are no longer helpful.

We will start exactly where you started, with the behaviour or situation that made you realize it was time to change. We will install the swish pattern that redirects your decision. To put it simply, we are telling your brain, 'Not that, this!' Then whenever that situation arises, a powerful new drive towards health will emerge to take you towards new, rewarding, healthy behaviour. The more you repeat the exercise, the stronger the new drive, as it creates new neural pathways associating the old stimulus with the desired new outcome.

THE SWISH

Practise this technique right now, and use it as often as you wish, whenever you have to make a decision about food or drink. Do this exercise somewhere where you can safely close your eyes and be undisturbed for two or three minutes. Keep your eyes closed throughout this exercise. If you'd like me to talk you through it, put on the CD.

1. Think now of the time you decided to use this book. What exactly was it for you about sugar that made you realize: 'It is time to change'? I would like you now to make a snapshot in your mind of the behaviour around sugar that made you want to use this book. Make the picture very clear. Now imagine putting that image to one side for a moment.

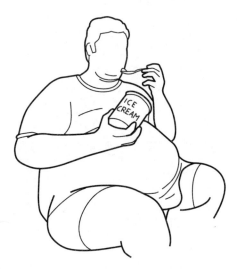

2. Create a picture of how you intend to be when you are back in control of your own appetite. See how you will look. You may have lost weight. You may be more relaxed. You may be fitter, you may be happier and more at ease. Take a little time to build that picture and fill in all the detail. Take a little while to enjoy it, then compress and shrink it down to a little dot way, way, away in the distance.

3. Bring back the picture of the behaviour you want to change. See it right in front of you.

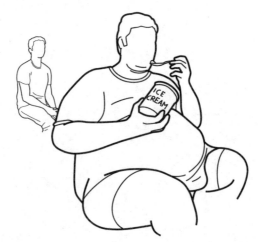

4.   Now imagine the picture of the healthy future accelerating towards you from that distant dot, getting bigger, brighter and clearer as it gets closer and closer until suddenly it smashes the old behaviour picture into a million pieces. Make the new, healthy picture big, bright and vivid and let it fill your field of vision. Enjoy the good feelings for a few moments.

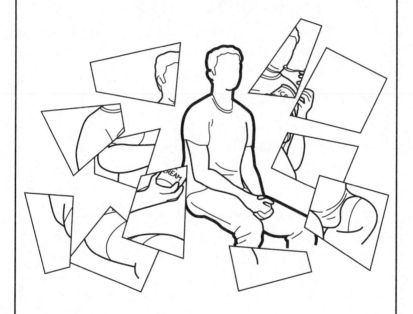

5.   Repeat steps 3 and 4 ten times, as fast as you can, keeping the images clear and distinct all the time.

Used with the written permission of Dr Richard Bandler

IN A NUTSHELL

- Sugar stops you feeling full

- Sugar-eaters are not in control

- Reset your 'fullness' signalling to restore your control

- Use the Swish to smash old sugar-eating habits

5

·

DO YOU KNOW HOW MUCH SUGAR YOU DRINK?

DO YOU KNOW HOW MUCH SUGAR YOU DRINK?

The sugarcane plant comes from South-east Asia. Sugar was first extracted and crystallized in India around 650AD. In the Middle Ages it was brought to Western Europe and sugar plantations were set up in Sicily, but sugar remained a rare and expensive luxury.

When Europeans colonized the Americas they took sugar cane with them. In the eighteenth century, a German scientist discovered how to extract sugar from sugar beet, and large-scale production was ordered by Napoleon fifty years later when his enemies were preventing ships from bringing cane sugar from the Americas.

When sugar was still a rare and expensive luxury, consumption was controlled by price. Only the very rich could afford sugar on a regular basis, and they paid for the privilege with dental caries and obesity. The huge increase in obesity, diabetes and heart disease in the twentieth century can be directly correlated to the fall in the cost of sugar, the massive increase in sugar consumption, and the widespread use of sugar in the industrialization of food and drink.

Sugar killer on the shelves

There is one more dangerous source of sugar on the supermarket shelves which has been passed off as a health hero for years: fruit juice. Adverts for fruit juice normally show one or both of two things: a delicious, shiny, fresh, ripe fruit, and a super healthy, slim model. Both, sadly, are misleading. Here is why.

Fruit

In fruit we find water, fibre, vitamins, and both sucrose (which is half fructose) and fructose itself. The water and the vitamins are good for you. The sucrose and the fructose are not good for you, but the fibre saves the day for two reasons. First, when you eat fruit the fibre makes you feel physically full. Even though we know the fructose won't tell your brain to stop, your stomach will fill up so the nerves in the stomach wall will signal your brain to stop eating. Secondly, the fibre lines your intestine, forming an extra barrier so that the fructose passes into your bloodstream more slowly and your liver can process more of it before it becomes overloaded.

The truth about juice

Fruit juice is basically fruit with all the fibre removed. It is water (good), vitamins (good), sucrose (bad) and fructose (bad). It has a reputation for health because of the vitamins, but without fibre to slow it down, the fructose and sucrose hit our bloodstream fast and hard. That is bad.

Much worse, however, is the fact that without the fibre we don't feel full. Our stomachs do not expand and tell our brain we have had enough because the water is quickly exported. We end up filling ourselves with far more sugar than we could possibly ingest if we were eating the whole fruit. It would be a struggle to eat one and half kilos of apples, but it is relatively easy to drink half a litre of apple juice.

Anyone can survive a glass of fruit juice on an occasional basis, but regular consumption of fruit juice means a regular battering with fructose. That makes people fat and increases the risk of heart attack. This may sound strange given that fruit and juice have both been marketed as healthy for decades, but the scientific reality is unequivocal.

Fruit is good for you.

Fruit juice is bad for you.

Another way to look at this is to understand that our bodies are perfectly evolved to digest naturally occurring foods, including fructose in seasonal fruit. It is only when we extract the sucrose and fructose and serve it without the protective fibre that it screws up our system.

Fruit juice is another reason why the standard American and British breakfast is such a disaster. For years people have had orange juice at breakfast because it was marketed as a healthy source of vitamin C. Vitamin C is great. But it is far better inside an orange, with all the useful and protective fibre.

Once you have installed all the techniques in this book, your sugar consumption will be dramatically lowered so you will be able to choose where and when you have sugar.

One glass of apple juice actually contains more sugar than the equivalent amount of cola, so you can certainly enjoy fruit juice from time to time, but you will think of it as a treat, like a dessert. You will no longer drink it without thinking.

Don't drink fruit juice. Eat fruit.

If you are thirsty, drink water or milk.

Smoothies

The modern version of fruit juice is the smoothie. Smoothies are mostly combinations of juiced fruit with yoghurt and other flavourings. Some have concentrated juice as an ingredient, which essentially means concentrated sugar. That healthy image can still conceal a whole heap of sugar. There are smoothies made with plain yoghurt and whole fruit, but it pays to be careful around smoothies, especially as blending chops up the fibres in fruit and makes them less effective inside your digestive system. As you consume less sugar you will become more sensitive, so your tongue will tell you when there is sugar in a smoothie. If there is, be careful!

Sugar-sweetened beverages

Let's look now at one of the great commercial success stories of the twentieth century: sweetened soda drinks. Supermarkets and convenience stores have shelves and shelves of drinks. Somewhere low down and inconvenient is the water and the milk. The other shelves are loaded with fizzy drinks, soft drinks, smoothies, energy drinks, flavoured milks, drinking yoghurt, organic drinks, juices and nectars. They are all loaded with sugar. Some of the worst are the ones with a reputation for healthiness like yoghurts and smoothies.

Scientists and doctors have been so concerned about drinks containing sugar that they have been doing research on them for over a decade. They write about them so much that they have an acronym, SSB, standing for Sugar Sweetened Beverages. I will just call them sodas or soft drinks.

Soft drinks are sugar and water, usually carbonated, with a pinch of flavouring. The average can of soft drink contains 35 grams of sugar. That's about eight teaspoons. That is 5 grams more than the total daily amount for an adult recommended by the UK government.

Many people grab a can of cola every lunchtime, or take one to drink as they walk from A to B, and they hardly think about it. They certainly don't think it is more than the entire recommended dose for an adult for a day. Actually there is good reason to believe that the recommended level is still too high, as studies have shown that just one soda per day leads to a significantly greater risk of heart disease than that of people who have no sodas at all.

Dealing with thirst

Soft drinks are sold as thirst-quenchers but many are designed to make you more likely to want another one. For example, most colas contain sugar, salt and caffeine. Caffeine is a diuretic. It makes you want to pee, and that depletes your water supply. Salt also makes you thirsty, but you can't taste the salt because it is hidden by the sugar. Being in liquid form, the sugar hits your bloodstream quickly. It causes a glucose spike and an insulin spike, so people have too much sugar and then too little. These factors all combine to make you more likely to want another cup of cola. They may have a nice taste and an attractive zing, but no soft drink quenches your thirst as well as water alone does.

Too much sugar

Research has shown that the more sodas a person drinks, the more likely they are to be overweight and the higher their risk of heart disease. The average American gets 30 per cent of their daily sugar consumption from sodas. We don't have exact figures for UK consumption and it is likely to be below that, but we are following close behind.

Sugar-laden beverages are doubly dangerous because they contain no fibre whatsoever. There is absolutely nothing to stop people drinking SSBs. The body does not register the fructose input because satiety is not triggered, so fat from the fructose is added on top of whatever food is eaten and registered.

Research has demonstrated that when children are given a soda before eating a fast-food meal, they eat more than they would otherwise. It is doubly fattening. It is not surprising that fast-food outlets promote colas and meal deals so heavily and it is not surprising we have an epidemic of childhood obesity.

Hot sugar

I stopped taking sugar in my tea and coffee after talking to Dr Ruden. I realized I didn't really pay attention to the sweetness of the drink, it was more that I felt it just wasn't such good tea or coffee without it. In fact, my taste buds had been blunted by my continuous sugar consumption.

I had a habit of taking two spoonfuls of sugar with each cup. So I carried on, but each day I scraped a little bit of sugar off the spoonful, so very gradually I reduced the amount I used. The difference was so small each day that my taste buds couldn't tell the difference, but within two weeks I had reduced my sugar usage to less than one-eighth of a spoonful, and importantly I was still enjoying my drinks. When I finally added no sugar at all, I still enjoyed them. You may find it useful to use this same trick.

Coffee shops always have sugar available to add to your drink, but I was astonished to find how much sugar was already included in some of the fancy drinks they sell. Caramel flavours, frappuccinos, chai lattes and iced coffees are often served with massive amounts of sugar already included. Sugar addicts drink them without any idea of how much sugar they contain. You don't need me to list the amounts of sugar – the internet is full of helpful posts giving the exact amounts. The key thought is this: if you don't know the precise ingredients in every drink you order, the chances are that it will contain sugar. If you don't know, ask.

But where is the fun?

OK, so now I have pointed out the dangers of some of the most popular beverages on the planet, what is left?

We have to remember that all of us buy these drinks for two reasons:

1.   **We are thirsty.**
2.   **We like them.**

We slake our thirst and get pleasure from these drinks. As you are going to drink less of them for a while, we need to make sure you can still quench your thirst and you can still have a lot of fun.

Thirst

The best drinks for quenching your thirst are water and milk. If they don't taste great, you weren't really, really thirsty. But many of us like sodas because we like the fizz and the sweetness. If you really like sodas you can get off sugar by drinking the sugar-lite or sugar-zero versions, which use artificial sweeteners. There is a growing body of research indicating that sweeteners may have problematic effects in the long-term so I can't recommend them as a permanent solution. However, if you find it difficult to stop drinking sodas straight away, they might help you as a temporary measure while you move away from sugar.

Fun

Some drinks taste nice. As we are not going to have that particular pleasure so often, let's find another way to feel good. So now, instead of one juice or soda that quenches your thirst a little bit and is a little bit of pleasure, you will have two actions. One which really quenches your thirst and another which really gives you a boost.

The following technique is adapted from a procedure used by all sections of the US military to stop feeling overwhelmed and regain resilience in battle conditions. When you stop drinking sugar it is important that you move beyond any feelings of deprivation. In the long-term you will enjoy feeling fitter and healthier and living a longer life, but you also need a way to feel super-good immediately.

1. **If you are really thirsty, drink water or milk.**
2. **If you want a real pick-me-up, use this technique and give yourself a bigger, richer boost.**

INSTANT FEEL GOOD

This technique connects you with your deeper, positive feelings. It focuses on the heart because the heart is like a second brain. It has nearly the same number of connections with the rest of the body as the brain itself, and when your heart is beating with a steady, strong, relaxed rhythm, your whole body feels relaxed and energized. The technique is deceptively simple and when practised regularly leads to significant improvements in health. Before you do this technique, please read through it and practise one step at a time slowly, so that when it comes time to do it, it's automatic. If you would like me to guide you through it, you can use the CD and do it with me.

You can use this technique whenever you feel you want a little boost or you imagine you would like a cola or a fruit juice or even a different sort of sugar. Practise now by imagining a situation like that, so that you can easily do it for real when you need it.

1. Imagine a situation where you think you want a soda, juice or sugar hit. Notice the feeling that prompts that desire.
2. Stop. Put your hand on your heart. If it is safe to do so, close your eyes. Take in a slow, deep breath for at least three seconds. You can measure that time by counting 1,001, 1,002, 1,003 in your head. Then, exhale at the same rate, again counting 1,001, 1,002, 1,003 in your head. This will slow down your breathing and reduce unconscious tightness in the

muscles in your chest. Swiftly this changes your physiology, reducing tension and altering your brain chemistry to promote the release of endorphins and serotonin.

3. As you notice your feelings change, bring to mind a person, place or thing that makes you feel good. Make a picture of that person, place or thing and enjoy looking at it until you feel a smile coming to your face. It doesn't have to be a big smile that someone else could see, you just need to keep looking until you feel your facial muscles begin to respond.

4. When you have felt that smile, imagine sending that picture to the back of your mind where it can continue to influence you at an unconscious level as you carry on with your day.

Use this technique whenever you notice a random thought about sugar and you will retrain your body to turn away from sugary drinks and food and to access your own happy chemicals.

IN A NUTSHELL

- One can of fizzy drink has more than the recommended adult daily sugar intake

- Stop drinking fruit juice, eat fresh fruit instead

- Quench your thirst with water or milk

- Use the Instant Feel Good technique to feel great

6

·

WINNING THE SUGAR BATTLE

WINNING THE SUGAR BATTLE

By the end of this chapter, you will know all about the bad things sugar does and you will be well on the way to restoring your control over sugar and your health. Remember this book is not primarily about weight, it is about health. But as you consume less sugar, you will lose weight along the way. Now, let's get the last of the bad news out of the way.

How sugar leads to diabetes

In the last chapter I explained that fructose causes insulin resistance so the pancreas has to produce more insulin to do the same job as before. That puts a strain on the pancreas. If this continues for years on end, the pancreas stops working. That is type 2 diabetes. If it is not properly managed, diabetes leads to kidney disease, heart disease, blindness and amputations. In 2016 there were twenty amputations a day in the UK as a direct result of diabetes.

Sugar leads to metabolic syndrome

Chronic sugar consumption and insulin resistance cause more than diabetes. High insulin and high blood sugar together cause high blood pressure. High levels of circulating fatty acids cause cardiovascular disease and obesity. All these diseases cluster together so often that doctors have given the phenomenon its own name: 'metabolic syndrome'.

Metabolic syndrome consists of high blood pressure, high blood sugar, high circulating triglycerides (from fatty acids) and excess fat around the waistline. It leads to cardiovascular disease, diabetes and further obesity.

Researchers have differing opinions about the sequencing and interaction of the different elements of metabolic syndrome but it is very clear that metabolic syndrome and insulin resistance occur together. It is also clear that chronic sugar consumption causes insulin resistance.

The top five killers

The top five causes of premature death in the UK are:

1. Cancer
2. Heart disease
3. Stroke
4. Lung disease
5. Liver disease

Apart from lung disease, which is correlated to smoking, all the others are linked to sugar. The risks of heart disease, stroke and liver disease are raised by insulin resistance.

Obesity increases the risk of the most common forms of cancer, and insulin resistance is now also being linked to higher risk of cancer. In short:

High sugar consumption is correlated to four of the top five causes of premature death.

Hidden danger

Metabolic syndrome is not confined to obese people. Researchers in the USA have estimated that up to 40 per cent of the population who are not obese may be suffering from metabolic syndrome.

Healthcare systems worldwide spend an absolute fortune on managing diabetes and cardiovascular disease. The numbers run into billions in every Western country. In recent years the rate of death from cardiovascular disease has in fact declined. That is not because people are more healthy, but because medicine has advanced to treat heart disease more effectively. Many people still die of heart attacks or strokes but many others survive and have to live with disability or pain and undergo expensive operations and treatment.

Sugar behaves like a drug

The final deadly icing on the cake is this: sugar behaves more like a drug than a nutrient. Ingesting sugar triggers the release of dopamine in a part of the brain called the nucleus accumbens, which is concerned with motivation and reward. Dopamine is a hormone with a myriad of effects including enjoyment, motivation and pleasure. Sugar triggers a reward feeling. That feeling makes people want more.

However, research has demonstrated that if dopamine is continually stimulated, the brain reduces the number of dopamine receptors so the dopamine effect is less powerful. That causes people to eat more sugar to get the same levels of reward.

Once people have eaten more than a certain amount of sugar, they go over the threshold of receptor reduction. Their behaviour changes. That is why sugar addicts find it so difficult to eat just half a bar of chocolate.

Doctors argue about whether sugar is addictive or mildly addictive or not addictive at all. Some studies have showed that rats preferred sugar water to cocaine, but that does not prove that humans would behave identically. I personally don't think the precise definition matters. We do know that the dopamine response is essentially the same response that is present in alcohol or cocaine addicts. Sugar not only messes up your satiety, it specifically makes you want more sugar.

Sugar unmasked

Now you have the whole picture:

- **Sugar switches off fullness signalling.**
- **Sugar turns directly to fat.**
- **Sugar triggers insulin resistance and hence heart disease and diabetes.**
- **Sugar behaves like an addictive drug in the brain and makes people want to eat more sugar.**

People who drink soft drinks or have a slice of cake are not choosing to poison themselves. They eat and drink sugary things because they taste nice. People get pleasure from sugar and that is a good thing. But there is a limit beyond which sugar is not a good thing.

A large amount of sugar is a very, very bad thing. Sugar takes over. It corrupts the natural control system. Realistically, obesity is not a choice. It happens to people who have lost control of their appetite. No one consciously chooses to increase their risk of cancer or heart disease. There can, of course, be other causes of metabolic syndrome and obesity, but in my opinion 95 times out of 100 the culprit is sugar.

Killer food

Sugar is the ultimate killer food, and it is all the more effective because it works extremely slowly. For moderate eaters of sugar, it can take two or three decades before it pulls the trigger for heart disease and diabetes. However, because some children now drink and eat huge and unprecedented amounts of sugar, we have an epidemic of childhood obesity and diabetes. Type 2 diabetes used to be called 'late-onset' diabetes. Doctors had to change the name to type 2 diabetes because they started to diagnose it in younger people and children.

Sugar thoughts do not belong to your conscious mind

Unconscious desires for sugar are caused by biochemical processes in your body. They do not come from your conscious mind. Chronic sugar consumption reduces the number of available dopamine receptors so the sugar addict ends up craving more sugar to release more dopamine. Worse still, after a while the dopamine does not trigger the reward feeling as strongly because as the receptors shut down, the reward effect decreases, leaving the motivation or craving effect intact.

The average sugar addict is completely unaware of this sequence of events. They just think, 'I'd like a cola' or 'I'd like to eat that.' They have no idea that their appetite has been taken over by sugar.

When sugar causes insulin resistance it continually inhibits satiety. This condition can be sustained by people eating relatively small daily amounts of sugar interspersed with larger binges. That means regardless of how much food is inside a person, they can still want more.

Sugar makes it possible to be overfed and still not satisfied. This is the nightmare in which far too many people are trapped. The body does not want or need food, but the control system is itself out of control.

Who is in charge?

If you are not malnourished and you are not hungry but you cannot resist drinking soft drinks or eating sugar, you are not in charge of your own behaviour. You may even imagine that the cravings or habits come from a 'bad' part of you, but I believe that is not true. I believe the craving does not really originate in you, good or bad. I believe that seeking sugar is a consequence of the corruption of your appetite. That may sound a bit extreme, but I would like to show you how you can prove to yourself it is true.

Random thoughts about sugar

In chapter one we looked at sugar cravings and I showed you how to destroy them. But as you will have seen, there are plenty of times when the desire for sugar is not a craving. It is more like a random or idle thought, but it happens so often and it seems so natural that it can lead to eating or drinking far more sugar than you wanted.

This sort of thinking is not particularly strong or compulsive, but it is frequent and repetitive. It might be as simple as 'I'm thirsty' or a casual whim, 'That would be nice.' It is characterized by a sense of unimportance, and often the thought is: 'A couple of biscuits don't matter', or 'I'll just have this to perk me up – tomorrow I must cut down.' However, although the thoughts and the actions seem trivial, their persistence sustains a continual low dose of sugar which, in the long-term, is deadly.

This continual grazing on sugary drinks and foods is such an ordinary activity that you might not even notice you are doing it. A good friend of mine was a couple of stones overweight and was complaining to me that he couldn't lose it even though he was very careful at mealtimes. I pointed out to him that whenever I saw him at work he always had a pastry or a can of soda in his hand. If we stopped at a petrol station he always bought a bar of chocolate when he paid for his fuel. It was such an everyday part of his routine he didn't think about it. I saw him a couple of months later and he was noticeably slimmer. I asked what he had done and the answer was literally, 'Nothing.' He had just stopped his habit of mindless grazing while he was at work, and now all he bought at petrol stations was petrol. One simple change was all he needed.

How to know when you are in control

You may or may not be grazing on sugar, but just to check, make a choice now. Say to yourself, 'For one month, I choose to eat less sugar. I will have no sugary drinks, no sweets, no desserts, no added sugar and no chocolate.'

If you are in charge of your brain, you will find that easy. You are totally in control of the amount of sugar you consume. You can put down this book immediately and live a happy, fulfilled, sugar-free life. Saying 'I will not eat sugar' for you is just like saying 'I will not eat cinnamon' or 'I'm giving up carrots this month'. It is just a matter of a simple decision about a certain food or flavour.

If, however, you find that your brain is very soon repeatedly and frequently crowded with ideas about eating sugar, about how refreshing cola is, or about how much you desire to eat chocolate, you will see that this is not your choice. If you suddenly have a change of opinion that claims this test is silly and it does not mean anything if you have a piece of cake, you will see that something has influenced your opinion.

You choose to eat less sugar. Suddenly your brain is full of ideas of consuming it in large quantities. That is the opposite of what you just chose. Where did those ideas come from? They came from the nucleus accumbens, which can no longer feel good without an excessive flood of dopamine. Your brain is seeking sugar in order to restore good feelings. Sugar has infiltrated your appetite and hijacked it.

A power struggle

This is a real battle. On one side is sugar and all the businesses that make money out of sugar. On the other side is me, you and your body's natural ability to be healthy. I will show you how we are going to win the battle.

Think of a time when you had a thought you might want to eat or drink something sugary. It may appear to be something trivial like, 'Oh, I'd like a biscuit' or 'I fancy a cola' or 'One glass of sweetened juice won't make a difference'. At other times it may feel intense, 'I really need a cola', or it may build over time and be accompanied by imagining the food or drink.

If you reflect on it, the situation in which those thoughts occur is usually one of these:

- **After an hour of vigorous exercise.**
- **When you see an advert.**
- **When you see a pack of biscuits or a can of cola or similar.**

- **When you feel stressed.**
- **A 'random' thought.**

After an hour of vigorous exercise

This is one of the few times when it is safe to eat or drink pretty much anything. Exercise builds muscles and when muscles are depleted they will take in a lot of energy. After exercise, muscles absorb more glucose, and insulin resistance is reduced. Often, of course, your body will tell you that you really need a proper meal after exercise, so of course the sensible thing is to eat a real meal. However, if you are planning another hour of exercise, your body will happily digest sugar in the form of biscuits or even sodas if you need energy now and you are going to carry on burning it up.

When you see an advert

Advertisements are psychological instruments designed to make you desire things. If it is a successful advertisement, that is what it will do. First, it draws your attention to the brand. Next, it associates good feelings with the brand. Then it implies that you will feel better – for example happier, stronger, more confident or more successful – when you use the product.

This psychological assault is launched by every advert you see. Many fail, but those that succeed can change the way we think. When researchers blind-tested two famous colas, respondents tended to prefer cola B. However, when respondents were told the brand, not only did they prefer cola A, but the researchers observed increased activity in the areas of the brain registering pleasure. The brand was so powerful it changed the location and intensity of brain activity.

It has also been demonstrated that our brains can respond to imagery in the same way as they do to a real object, so food advertisements often have luscious photos of the product to make us imagine we are hungry. Hence just seeing an advert can stimulate a desire.

When you see a pack of biscuits or a can of cola or similar

Advertisements implant associations with positive feelings so that they will be activated next time you see the product. The logo is the link between the feeling generated by the advertising and the product, so there is an effect at the psychological level.

When you feel stressed

Eating can reduce the symptoms of stress. No one likes to feel uncomfortable and one of the easiest ways to change how we feel is to distract ourselves with a simple pleasure. Sugary snacks are a simple pleasure. People also use them to give themselves a little break. Some people have jobs that are consistently stressful and develop a habit of using sugar as a little break and stress-reliever every day.

We know that eating can temporarily reduce the symptoms

of stress, but eating does not cure it. Stress is a psychological problem and it is better addressed with a psychological cure.

A 'random' thought

A thought can appear to be random because it does not arise from your consciousness. It is not random, but the cause is invisible to the conscious mind. We cannot feel the reduction in dopamine receptors in our brain. All we feel is a sense of lack. We also have both conscious and unconscious knowledge of what alleviates that lack. The reduction in dopamine receptors caused by sugar causes us to crave sugar. The supposedly 'random' thought has been sent from the deeper level of your brain and just pops out when you are a bit bored or not fully absorbed in a specific task. It is not random. It was sent by sugar.

Real hunger

Of these five situations, only one of them is a suitable time to eat sugar. After vigorous exercise there is a genuine need for nourishment, and while sugar is not the best possible choice it is certainly a reasonable option.

False hunger

In the other four situations, the driver is not hunger but an emotional state or a psychological trigger. If a person eats sugar in any of these other circumstances, they get a short moment of pleasure and relief at the cost of long-term damage. They do not achieve long-term health or control. Chronic sugar addicts who have become overweight never feel real hunger, but keep eating because they never feel full.

The key to controlling sugar is psychological.

Regaining control

When you reduce your sugar intake below a certain point, your natural homeostasis, or balance mechanism, is restored. Idle thoughts and cravings fade rapidly and soon disappear entirely. Your appetite works correctly again. You can eat food and stop eating when you have had enough. You basically forget about sugar until on a special occasion you are offered a treat. You simply think less about sugar-laced foods and you don't feel that you are missing out.

If your sugar habit was stronger than you realized, it is probably because you were unaware you were continually topping up your sugar levels.

However, if you have had a habit of significant daily sugar consumption, it takes two to three days for your body to readjust so that the cravings noticeably diminish. During that time, you must use the hypnosis CD and all the techniques in this book diligently to minimize discomfort as you reset your appetite.

Each person has a different threshold and there is no practical way to predict it objectively.

You will discover your own threshold by reducing your sugar intake until:

- **You are eating and drinking no high-sugar products at all.**
- **You can go three days with minimal sugar with no effort.**
- **You feel that sugar/chocolate/soft drinks are options you can happily do without.**

I will show you exactly how to do this below. You don't have to do it overnight. Some people take one day, others take one or two weeks. You don't have to go any faster than is practical and comfortable for you.

When you genuinely feel that sugar is an option – in other words, an optional pleasure not a random thought, a whim, a need or a craving – you are free to consume sugar as a treat.

HOW TO STAY IN YOUR SAFE ZONE

We want to make sure that in the future you can consume safe amounts of sugar and really enjoy it without triggering random desires for more sugar or getting caught in the trap of overconsumption. You need to discover how much you can consume and not trigger cravings afterwards. This is your safe zone. Finding your safe zone is a bit like finding out how much alcohol you can drink without feeling bad the next day. Just as with alcohol there are degrees of impairment, so with sugar there are levels of craving. With sugar even random thoughts are dangerous. You may find, for example, that you can share a bar of chocolate with a friend over a coffee and simply forget about sugar for the rest of the week.

Each of us is different and it is impossible for me to predict how much sugar you can safely and enjoyably eat and how often you can do so. The best way for you to find out is by careful observation.

1. Make a note in your journal of the times when you experience sugar cravings or 'random' thoughts about sugar, such as when you hear your mind making up excuses to eat sugar, or a thought pops up like 'One such-and-such won't make a difference'. As you use this book and the CD, continue to make notes as the days pass and notice the downward trend.

2. Make a note of the first day on which you find that you have no random desires for sugar and no cravings. Keep making notes until you have three days in a row in which you have no random desires for sugar and no cravings.

3. Carry on as before and wait until someone else offers you something sugary, for example, a slice of cake at a birthday party, or a fruit-juice-based cocktail. Accept the treat and enjoy it.

4. Keep track of your own reactions over the next day or so. If you have no cravings or random desires for sugar, you are still in your safe zone.

5. Every time you choose to accept some sugar hereafter, make a note of your own responses over the next day or two. As soon as you notice the reappearance of random thoughts about having some sugar, you have found the threshold of your danger zone. This is your upper limit. Use the Craving Buster (page 39) on all your sugar thoughts or cravings.

6. Now you know that you can eat just less than this amount and you will be free from sugar thoughts and cravings, in control of your appetite, and don't need to make any special efforts at all. If you accidentally go over your limit, use the techniques in this book again to re-establish control and recalibrate your appetite.

7. Continue to actively monitor your own responses because over time your safe range can change. Your body is a living, organic system that changes over time and is responsive to the environment. If idle thoughts about sugar resurface, it is a signal to cut down a little until you are completely relaxed around food again and you feel free to say yes or no to sugar, and when you say yes to enjoy it fully.

UN-SUGAR SPOTTING

I sometimes pass the time in shops and restaurants by playing a game I used to call 'Sugar spotting'. Actually it should be called 'Un-sugar spotting' because the way to win is to find products that *don't* have sugar in them.

In the supermarket 75 per cent of products contain sugar. That is three out of four. So it is more difficult to find things *without* sugar hidden in them than it is to find products *with* sugar.

When you play the game for a while you discover that sugar is hidden in surprising places and surprising amounts. You probably know that tomato ketchup contains sugar, but did you know that one tablespoon of ketchup contains one teaspoonful of sugar? That's a lot. What about salad dressing? That sounds healthy, doesn't it? Actually most ready-made salad dressings contain sugar too. Flavoured milks and sweetened yoghurts also have way too much sucrose.

The most common giveaway sign that a product contains sugar is 'low-fat'. Taking fat out of products spoils the taste, so many products have added sugar to make up for it.

Next time you go shopping with a friend or partner or child, play 'Un-sugar spotting'. When you nominate a product, the other one has to check the ingredients label to see if there is sugar in it.

You will find it's there most of the time, even though it can hide under a different name.

SUGAR NAMES

Any box, bottle or can, any sauce, ready meal or frozen food has a three-in-four chance of containing sugar. Pretty much all commercially available drinks, apart from water and milk, contain sugar. Manufacturers try to disguise sugar by using more than fifty different names. Here are some of them, and you may find even more.

- Agave nectar
- Barbados sugar
- Barley malt
- Barley malt syrup
- Beet sugar
- Brown sugar
- Buttered syrup
- Cane juice
- Cane juice crystals
- Cane sugar
- Caramel
- Carob syrup
- Castor sugar
- Coconut palm sugar
- Coconut sugar
- Confectioner's sugar
- Corn sweetener
- Corn syrup
- Corn syrup solids
- Date sugar
- Dehydrated cane juice
- Demerara sugar
- Dextrin
- Dextrose
- Evaporated cane juice
- Fructose
- Fruit juice
- Fruit juice concentrate
- Golden sugar
- Golden syrup
- Grape sugar
- HFCS (High-Fructose Corn Syrup)
- Honey

- Icing sugar
- Invert sugar
- Malt syrup
- Maltodextrin
- Maltol
- Maltose
- Mannose
- Maple syrup
- Molasses
- Muscovado sugar
- Palm sugar
- Raw sugar
- Refiner's syrup
- Rice syrup
- Saccharose
- Sorghum syrup
- Sucrose
- Sweet sorghum
- Syrup
- Treacle
- Turbinado sugar
- Yellow sugar

Kicking sugar out

After one week of un-sugar spotting and finding different names for sugar, you will also be able to see that in your own daily life there are particular times and places in which you are most vulnerable to consuming sugar.

We all have routines, and sugar may be built into them without our conscious awareness. Everyday items such as breakfast cereal, orange juice, tomato ketchup and processed foods all add up to a cascade of sugar, and all of them are just small items in a daily routine.

When we interrupt that routine, we displace the cues for eating and we can dislodge large amounts of sugar from our daily life.

Un-sugar spotting will have shown you many of the places where you personally come across sugar, so you are now ready to make some changes. These changes can be very small and very simple but they will add up to a big and healthy change.

ROUTINE DISRUPTION

Do this exercise after you have been filling in the journal for at least a week.

1. Look at your journal for the first week of this system and notice the top five usual times and places where you are at risk of eating or drinking sugar. For example, you may have had a habit of drinking orange juice for breakfast or a caramel latte at 11 a.m. Some people snack on biscuits at the office, eat chocolate when they are driving or have an 'energy drink' at the gym.

2. For each of the top five times or places that you were consuming sugar, design a small change in your routine. For example, if you had an orange juice with breakfast, change the time you have breakfast or just change the position you sit at the table. If you normally picked up a flavoured coffee in the morning, buy it without the sugar flavouring. If you don't like that, walk in a different direction and buy a piece of fresh fruit instead. If you were used to an energy drink after a workout, take a bottle of plain or sparkling water and a banana and have them instead.

3. Introduce these changes into your life at your own pace. They may seem small, even petty, but they will add up to a massive change. Some people introduce all the changes on one day, others go more slowly. If you feel they are too difficult and irritating, then you probably need to make them even more, but you can make them very slowly. You could do just one per day, or even take three days to get used to one change before you add another. There are many ways to get this right, so long as each day, at whatever speed, you are changing your routine to exclude sugar.

Warnings

Once you have completed using this book, you will be in charge of your sugar intake and you can choose to consume sugar on your own terms. However, if you re-experience cravings, that is an alarm bell which tells you that sugar has invaded your control system again and you need to avoid it for three days to re-establish control.

You may not experience cravings at all, but you will notice you approach the edge of your safe zone when you find thoughts occurring like 'Oh, one extra piece doesn't matter' or 'Well, I'm not actually fat, so I can have another treat'. The moment you find your mind making up excuses is the moment it has been influenced by a craving. If your choice is genuinely free, you need no excuses. The excuses are a sign that you are approaching the danger zone.

You are most likely to find, after using this book, that 'warning' cravings and excuses are far weaker than the old habit or compulsion, so you need to be quite alert to spot them and to respond. If your 'warning' cravings are intense, and for some people they are, especially early on, it is much easier to spot them, and as soon as you do so you have to apply the Craving Buster (see page 39) immediately to control them.

IN A NUTSHELL

- Sugar is linked to four of the top five causes of premature death

- Sugar behaves like an addictive drug

- Sugar infects your appetite mechanism

- Establish your Safe Zone and stay within it so you can trust your appetite again

- Use Routine Disruption to remove sugar from your daily life

7
·
A BRIGHTER
FUTURE

A BRIGHTER FUTURE

As I worked on this book, something puzzled me more and more. Our bodies are astonishingly efficient machines that have evolved over tens of thousands of years. How come they have such a disastrous response to fructose? Then one day I thought: Maybe it's not a disaster. Maybe the way we metabolize fructose is an adaption that helped us to survive.

Before people learned to extract the juice of the sugar cane, fructose was found only in fruit (and in honey, which was not easy to obtain). Fruit tends to be ripe, sweet and full of fructose in summer and autumn, just before the winter months when food is scarce. Fructose converts to fat very efficiently so fruit is a treasure chest of energy. I believe we evolved a specific metabolism for dealing with fructose in order to get as much energy on board as possible when fruit was in season and to store it to get us through the winter.

There is nothing wrong with our bodies. We are perfectly suited to an environment where sugar is rare and seasonal, but in the last hundred years our food environment has changed so fast and so drastically that we are now in mortal danger.

Added sugar

Sugar is added to almost all manufactured food and drinks, and people consume it day in day out, all year long. Most people have no idea that so many of the products they buy every week contain sugar because the sweet taste might not be obvious. There are thousands of products containing sugar that are based on traditional recipes that originally had no sugar in them. Traditional or home-made pasta sauce, yoghurt and pizza don't contain sugar. Almost all the versions that are made in factories do. Sugar is very useful to manufacturers as a preservative and flavour enhancer. It is not at all useful to us.

Convenience

People buy ready meals and packaged food because they are convenient. They are not aware of the amount of sugar they are buying. After a busy working day lots of people don't want to cook, and they certainly don't want to cook twice, once for the children and again for themselves. It is easier to open a packet and use the microwave.

The disadvantage is that short-term convenience comes at a cost of a long-term risk of disease, which is seriously inconvenient. In Britain, in 2015, one in three of our children were too heavy and one in five dangerously so. Those kids are not heading for a healthy life.

Increasing numbers of adults and children are being diagnosed with diabetes, which is also inconvenient. Diabetics have to manage their condition all day, every day. If they don't, they risk the further inconvenience of heart disease, blindness or amputations.

In the end, as the old saying goes, there is no such thing as a free lunch. As you move away from sugar you will find at first that you spend a bit more time finding foods without sugar. You may start cooking differently or cooking more often. You may spend an extra minute or two peeling fruit and having to wash your hands afterwards instead of just opening a carton of juice. Of course, when you have established your new routines and found better food to buy or cook, it won't seem like an effort at all. You may discover you enjoy it more.

You will find yourself making lots of small or even tiny changes like this as you take more control of your appetite and move away from sugar. All those little extra efforts each day now will be repaid with years of good health.

New perceptions

As you use the techniques in this book, many of you will have noticed that you have started seeing food differently and are spotting the sugar in all the food it contaminates. You will start to see the dull and dangerous reality of mass-produced food and drink. You will notice more and more often how sweet foods make you want more, but ten minutes later you are still not satisfied.

Have you ever wondered why there are so many foods

that come in a can or box or bag with a picture on it? They hide the stuff you are buying because it looks drab and boring. Confectionery brands have bright, colourful logos. Underneath the wrapping, they all look the same: small brown bars.

The modern supermarket is the opposite of an old-fashioned food market. Many of us only see a fresh food market when we go on holiday. There are mountains of beautiful shiny fruit and vegetables. There are colourful herbs and spices. There are slightly scary-looking lumps of meat and sometimes even live fish in bowls of water. I personally would not know how to cook most of it, but I know I'm looking at real food. In the average supermarket what I mostly see is cans, boxes, bags and ready meals. And now I know that three out of four products I'm seeing in the supermarket are stuffed with added sugar.

We can change the world

There is a simple, powerful way to change what food and beverage companies make. We just stop buying their junk. It won't happen overnight, but it will happen. When you stop buying it, they will stop making it because it will lose them money.

At the same time, you have to eat and drink and enjoy life, so you will end up buying better produce, eating more fresh fruit or veg and drinking more water or milk. The companies that get good food to you will prosper. Those that don't will die. So, in the end, we have the power to change our own environments.

Labelling

Food manufacturers use all sorts of additives to stop their products from spoiling and to con us into buying more. They have to put the names of some of those additives on the labels, but they are not yet forced to tell us how much added sugar there is, so they don't.

And they are very experienced in presenting the facts in the most flattering light possible. They know how to use 'serving sizes' to obscure the total amount of sugar in their products, and how to add sugar to items to make them appear low-fat.

They also know how to fool people by highlighting one element to distract from another. For example, a cereal might have a big flash reading 'Wholegrain' or 'Multi-vitamin' to stop you paying attention to the fact that 25 per cent of it is sugar.

The simplest guide to labelling is to remember that if it needs a label, there is a three-in-four chance it is risky already. If it comes in a box, a can or a bottle it has been manufactured down to a cost, not up to a quality. Try to buy as much of your food as possible in its simplest form, then you know what you are getting. If you buy butter, you know what it is. If you buy milk, it's milk. If you buy peas, you get peas. Eating more simply for a while will help to re-educate your taste buds. If you want to get fancy, you can try cooking more stuff at home and making things like pasta sauces from scratch. You might even be surprised to find it is cheaper, it tastes good and you feel good about making it yourself.

You know what to do and where to go

You do not need to try to remove all sugar from your life. As you practise these techniques and complete the journal, you will discover your personal safe zone in which you are free to enjoy sugar.

I know many people find it difficult to believe they can actually enjoy life more without sugar, so we have one more technique to restore and reinforce your ability to feel satisfied, fulfilled and happy without any need for sugar at all.

Happiness

Food is not just about satisfying hunger. Food is about pleasure. We all enjoy eating food and sharing a meal with friends and family. It is one of the great joys of life. I am determined that as you eat less sugar you should enjoy all of your life more than ever before. You will enjoy a longer, healthier, fitter life, but I also want you to enjoy your food more. I want you to feel truly satisfied by truly delicious meals.

It is also time to reclaim all the beautiful human emotions that have been used and demeaned by drink and food advertising. You don't need sugary, tooth-rotting fizz to make friends. You don't need fast-food junk to show your children you love them. You don't need an ice cream to create a romantic moment with your partner.

It is time to separate sugar brands from the feelings they have evoked to make people feel better about their products. Love, kindness and happiness do not belong to branded foods. They are feelings we generate in our own lives by our own presence, kindness, care and compassion.

The big scientific breakthrough

If you have read some of my previous books you will know about the astounding power of Havening, a deceptively simple process developed by Dr Ronald Ruden, which eliminates post-traumatic stress disorder and resets the biochemical landscape of the brain.

Havening is a sequence of touches and eye movements that breaks down the neural pathways in which trauma is encoded. Havening allows cognitive memory to function properly but it severs the automated link to traumatic feeling. Severe cases of post-traumatic stress can be massively improved or completely cured in a single session of Havening.

Dr Ruden and I were part of the research team at King's College London led by Professor Neil Greenberg that focused on alleviating post-traumatic stress disorder. We have continued to develop Havening over the last few years.

Changing feelings

We know many people eat sugar to change the way they feel. Some people do this without noticing they are doing it. Dr Ruden and I have found we can use Havening to establish a sense of well-being that eliminates this need to change feelings. When confidence, relaxation and control are established, individuals no longer need to medicate themselves with food.

In this development, Havening 'locks in' a positive neural circuit associated with the positive visualization. In very young infants, huge amounts of information flood the brain through the senses and the new human being has to make sense of it all. This organizing principle is supported by delta-wave activity.

Infants have been shown to spend a great deal of time in slow-wave sleep, and thus have more delta-wave activity. In fact, delta waves are the predominant wave forms of infants. In adults, the delta wave is seen only in slow-wave sleep. Dr Ruden believes that it is this electrical wave, produced by Havening Touch after activation of an emotional memory, that allows us to encode the new information.

HAVENING: A NEW SENSE OF WELL-BEING

We can use this technique now to reinforce your freedom from sugar. Read this technique through completely before you do it. Do this only at a time and place where you can concentrate totally and completely on this technique. Whenever it is possible, use the CD and do it as I talk you through it.

1. Put your left hand on your right shoulder and your right hand on your left shoulder and begin to stroke the outside of your arms gently and firmly, producing the calming effect of delta waves.

2. Now imagine watching a full-colour movie, directly in front of you, of a you that is free from desires of sugar and is full of confidence and completely at ease. The new you looks straight past the sweet counter, smiles and waves away the dessert trolley and never needs sugar in tea or coffee. In this movie you are happy, relaxed and smiling.

3. Keep watching and see a situation arise that used to be stressful and watch yourself deal with it firmly and successfully, staying confident and relaxed.

4. Enjoy looking at yourself handling things well, keeping your good humour and your power.

5. Keep doing the Havening Touch, stroking the sides of your arms, and when the movie looks really, really good, imagine floating into the healthier, happier you. See through the eyes

of your happier, healthier self, hear through the ears of your healthier, happier self and feel how good you feel.

Do this exercise every day for seven days and then use it as often as you wish thereafter. If you want to find out more detail about the science behind Havening and other ways in which it can be used, visit www.havening.org.

USE THE JOURNAL AND ALL THE TECHNIQUES

Over the next week I need you to rehearse and practise all the techniques you have learned in this book. Some you will find very easy; some you may find more difficult. Please concentrate particularly on those you do not yet find easy. Practice now will really help over the next month.

Each one of us is starting from a different place. Even people whose livers are almost burned out can recover to spectacular good health when they stop eating excess sugar. The human body is wonderful at repairing itself, so long as we give it a chance.

Some of you don't eat confectionery; some of you don't drink fruit juice; some of you don't drink colas. Each of us already has some areas free from sugar, and others where we will be making changes. Although those changes will be rapid, you can be sure that as you use the techniques the change will be no faster than is right for you.

The first seven days will set the course for the reduction in your sugar intake. During the following thirty days you will stabilize a low level of sugar intake that will last for a longer, healthier lifetime.

Reread and reuse the book and CD as much as you want and as often as you need.

PASSIONS

I have written this book because I am passionate about this subject. For me, this is the missing piece of the jigsaw I have been working on for twenty-five years. I have helped millions of people to lose weight, but I have never been completely satisfied because I was not able to help everyone who was truly willing.

When I first looked at weight loss twenty-five years ago, I initially suggested that people avoid sugar. Although at that time I did not know the scientific facts, I could see that many of the people who had problems with their weight ate a lot of sugar. However, I could also see that food-controlling diets were a disaster so I decided to focus completely on the psychological side.

My instinct that we need to restore our sense of fullness was correct. It is only in the last ten to fifteen years that it has become clear that fructose not only causes obesity and disease but also interferes with the satiety or fullness signalling.

Your fabulous future

Now that we understand the problem, I want to share the solution as widely as possible. I want you, and your family, and your friends and neighbours, to be part of a movement that puts sugar back where it belongs.

Sugar is like champagne. If someone drinks champagne every day, pours it on their cereal, adds it to shepherd's pie and mixes it in their milk, it is not special and it is not enjoyable and it spoils the taste of everything else.

Sugar, like champagne, should be a special treat for a special occasion. When you have sugar from this moment onwards, I want you to enjoy every gram of it. I also want you to enjoy the rest of your food just as much. By the time you have completed your journal, you will know how to eat and drink to stay in your safe zone and be free from cravings. Your days of playing 'Un-sugar spotting' will have shown you how to avoid buying sugar by mistake and your new routines will have removed the worst sources of sugar in your old life.

Perfectly imperfect

You don't have to be perfect on your path to freedom from sugar. I'm sure you will make a few mistakes and drink or eat sugar in a moment of absent-mindedness or by accident. Don't worry. Each time you do that it will be more and more noticeable, and every technique you practise will strengthen the structure of your new, free life.

IN A NUTSHELL

- Your body works fine. The problem is sugar

- The more good food you buy, the more good food they will provide

- Use Havening to 'lock in' the healthy version of your future

- Use your journal every day to track your progress

SUGAR
CONTROL
JOURNAL

SUGAR CONTROL JOURNAL

Research has shown us that writing down our commitments, and keeping written track of progress, leads to quicker and more profound changes.

As soon as you use this journal you will start to benefit. Some days you may want to write a lot, some days you will be done in less than a minute. That is fine. Just check in every day to make a note of which techniques you use or practise, and notice how each day you move further away from sugar and into a richer, healthier, balanced life.

By the way, nobody ever gets it perfect straight away. If you miss something, don't worry. Just carry on and fill it in as soon as you can. You will soon build the habit of writing for just a minute a day and you will notice the benefits very quickly.

Techniques

DAY 1

START NOW

**My current sugar consumption across
all kinds of food and drink**

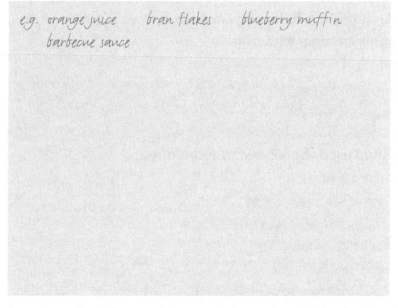

e.g. orange juice   bran flakes   blueberry muffin
barbecue sauce

*Don't worry if you don't track down every gram of sugar immediately.
You can add to the list later. Now reread what you've written and
underline the top five items, places or times where you feel you are
consuming too much sugar.*

Today I used the Mind-programming Technique CD yes

DAY 2

Make sure you have at least one breakfast this week as free from sugar as possible.

Is today a healthy breakfast day?   yes

I noticed the following cravings or random sugar thoughts:

And I used the following techniques:

Craving Buster   yes

Defence against Advertising   yes

Program Your Mind for a Healthy Future   yes

The Swish   yes

Instant Feel Good   yes

Havening: A New Sense of Well-being   yes

I noticed these positive changes:

Today I used the Mind-programming Technique CD   yes

DAY 3

Is today a healthy breakfast day?   yes

**I noticed the following cravings or
random sugar thoughts:**

And I used the following techniques:

Craving Buster   yes

Defence against Advertising   yes

Program Your Mind for a Healthy Future   yes

The Swish   yes

Instant Feel Good   yes

Havening: A New Sense of Well-being   yes

I noticed these positive changes:

Today I used the Mind-programming Technique CD yes

DAY 4

Is today a healthy breakfast day?   yes

I noticed the following cravings or random sugar thoughts:

And I used the following techniques:

Craving Buster   yes

Defence against Advertising   yes

Program Your Mind for a Healthy Future   yes

The Swish   yes

Instant Feel Good   yes

Havening: A New Sense of Well-being   yes

I noticed these positive changes:

Today I used the Mind-programming Technique CD   yes

DAY 5

If you have not started yet, today is a good day to begin to Reset Your Fullness Signal. Turn to page 87 and follow the instructions there.

Is today a healthy breakfast day?   yes

I noticed the following cravings or random sugar thoughts:

And I used the following techniques:

Craving Buster   yes

Defence against Advertising   yes

Program Your Mind for a Healthy Future   yes

The Swish   yes

Instant Feel Good   yes

Havening: A New Sense of Well-being   yes

I noticed these positive changes:

Today I used the Mind-programming Technique CD yes

DAY 6

Is today a healthy breakfast day?   yes

I noticed the following cravings or random sugar thoughts:

And I used the following techniques:

Craving Buster   yes

Defence against Advertising   yes

Program Your Mind for a Healthy Future   yes

The Swish   yes

Instant Feel Good   yes

Havening: A New Sense of Well-being   yes

I noticed these positive changes:

Today I used the Mind-programming Technique CD   yes

DAY 7

Is today a healthy breakfast day?   yes

I noticed the following cravings or random sugar thoughts:

And I used the following techniques:

Craving Buster   yes

Defence against Advertising   yes

Program Your Mind for a Healthy Future   yes

The Swish   yes

Instant Feel Good   yes

Havening: A New Sense of Well-being   yes

I noticed these positive changes:

Today I used the Mind-programming Technique CD   yes

DAY 8

Congratulations! You have practised the techniques for one week now. Look back and check whether you skipped any. If so, that's fine, but do the missing ones now to catch up.

Is today a healthy breakfast day?   yes

I noticed the following cravings or random sugar thoughts:

I used these techniques to improve my health:

I noticed these positive changes:

DAY 9

Now it is time to start to use the Sugar Routine Disruption. Turn to page 130 and follow the instructions there.

Go for at least two breakfasts this week as free from sugar as possible.

Is today a healthy breakfast day?   yes

I noticed the following cravings or random sugar thoughts:

I used these techniques to improve my health:

I noticed these positive changes:

DAY 10

Is today a healthy breakfast day? yes

I noticed the following cravings or random sugar thoughts:

I used these techniques to improve my health:

I noticed these positive changes:

DAY 11

Is today a healthy breakfast day?   yes

**I noticed the following cravings or
random sugar thoughts:**

I used these techniques to improve my health:

I noticed these positive changes:

DAY 12

Is today a healthy breakfast day?   yes

**I noticed the following cravings or
random sugar thoughts:**

I used these techniques to improve my health:

I noticed these positive changes:

DAY 13

Is today a healthy breakfast day?   yes

I noticed the following cravings or
random sugar thoughts:

I used these techniques to improve my health:

I noticed these positive changes:

DAY 14

Is today a healthy breakfast day?   yes

**I noticed the following cravings or
random sugar thoughts:**

I used these techniques to improve my health:

I noticed these positive changes:

DAY 15

Is today a healthy breakfast day?   yes

**I noticed the following cravings or
random sugar thoughts:**

I used these techniques to improve my health:

I noticed these positive changes:

DAY 16

Now you are getting control back. Aim for at least three breakfasts this week as free from sugar as possible.

Is today a healthy breakfast day?   yes

I noticed the following cravings or random sugar thoughts:

I used these techniques to improve my health:

I noticed these positive changes:

DAY 17

Is today a healthy breakfast day?   yes

I noticed the following cravings or
random sugar thoughts:

I used these techniques to improve my health:

I noticed these positive changes:

DAY 18

Is today a healthy breakfast day?   yes

**I noticed the following cravings or
random sugar thoughts:**

I used these techniques to improve my health:

I noticed these positive changes:

DAY 19

Is today a healthy breakfast day?   yes

I noticed the following cravings or random sugar thoughts:

I used these techniques to improve my health:

I noticed these positive changes:

DAY 20

Is today a healthy breakfast day?   yes

I noticed the following cravings or
random sugar thoughts:

I used these techniques to improve my health:

I noticed these positive changes:

DAY 21

Is today a healthy breakfast day?   yes

**I noticed the following cravings or
random sugar thoughts:**

I used these techniques to improve my health:

I noticed these positive changes:

DAY 22

Is today a healthy breakfast day?   yes

I noticed the following cravings or random sugar thoughts:

I used these techniques to improve my health:

I noticed these positive changes:

DAY 23

Enjoy being in control. Have at least four breakfasts this week as free from sugar as possible.

Is today a healthy breakfast day?   yes

I noticed the following cravings or random sugar thoughts:

I used these techniques to improve my health:

I noticed these positive changes:

DAY 24

Is today a healthy breakfast day?   yes

**I noticed the following cravings or
random sugar thoughts:**

I used these techniques to improve my health:

I noticed these positive changes:

DAY 25

Is today a healthy breakfast day?   yes

I noticed the following cravings or random sugar thoughts:

I used these techniques to improve my health:

I noticed these positive changes:

DAY 26

Is today a healthy breakfast day?   yes

I noticed the following cravings or
random sugar thoughts:

I used these techniques to improve my health:

I noticed these positive changes:

DAY 27

Is today a healthy breakfast day?   yes

I noticed the following cravings or
random sugar thoughts:

I used these techniques to improve my health:

I noticed these positive changes:

DAY 28

Is today a healthy breakfast day?   yes

**I noticed the following cravings or
random sugar thoughts:**

I used these techniques to improve my health:

I noticed these positive changes:

DAY 29

Is today a healthy breakfast day?   yes

**I noticed the following cravings or
random sugar thoughts:**

I used these techniques to improve my health:

I noticed these positive changes:

DAY 30

There comes a point with any new habit when it is easier to do it than not do it. So, let's keep the momentum going and make sure you have at least five breakfasts this week as free from sugar as possible.

Is today a healthy breakfast day?   yes

I noticed the following cravings or random sugar thoughts:

I used these techniques to improve my health:

I noticed these positive changes:

DAY 31

Is today a healthy breakfast day?   yes

I noticed the following cravings or
random sugar thoughts:

I used these techniques to improve my health:

I noticed these positive changes:

DAY 32

Is today a healthy breakfast day?   yes

I noticed the following cravings or
random sugar thoughts:

I used these techniques to improve my health:

I noticed these positive changes:

DAY 33

Is today a healthy breakfast day? yes

I noticed the following cravings or random sugar thoughts:

I used these techniques to improve my health:

I noticed these positive changes:

DAY 34

Is today a healthy breakfast day?   yes

I noticed the following cravings or
random sugar thoughts:

I used these techniques to improve my health:

I noticed these positive changes:

DAY 35

Is today a healthy breakfast day?   yes

I noticed the following cravings or
random sugar thoughts:

I used these techniques to improve my health:

I noticed these positive changes:

DAY 36

Is today a healthy breakfast day?   yes

I noticed the following cravings or random sugar thoughts:

I used these techniques to improve my health:

I noticed these positive changes:

DAY 37

Now you are ready to have at least six breakfasts a week as free from sugar as possible.

Is today a healthy breakfast day?   yes

**I noticed the following cravings or
random sugar thoughts:**

I used these techniques to improve my health:

I noticed these positive changes:

REVIEW

Congratulations! Pat yourself on the back. Your brilliant achievement will give you a long life and keep you healthy and happier. Sadly, there will be a few people who did not make it to the end of this journal. You did! That is what separates you from the rest. You are a winner.

Look back now over the last 37 days and review all the positive trends you can identify in your journal.

If you feel there is still more progress to be made, buy a notebook and continue this journal. Continue using all the tools of this system until you feel happy and confident with your new lifestyle, your new relationship with food, and a small, safe and fully appreciated amount of sugar.

If you now feel healthy and happy with your new habits, keep using the techniques and mind-programming whenever you feel you need them.

If you want to know a bit more about the science and the politics behind sugar in the food industry, look at the further reading section which follows here.

FURTHER READING

The leading clinician and researcher in the battle against sugar in the United States is Dr Robert Lustig. His book is a comprehensive review of the metabolism of sugar and the damage it does. *Fat Chance: The hidden truth about sugar, obesity and disease*, Fourth Estate, London 2014

Dr John Yudkin's book, first published in 1972 and revised in 1986, is a clear and careful presentation of the dangers of sugar, and records early pressure from the sugar industry to suppress his work. *Pure, White and Deadly: How sugar is killing us and what we can do to stop it*, reissued by Penguin Books, London 2012

David Gillespie is an Australian lawyer who lost 40 kilos simply by cutting sugar out of his diet. His book documents his research into the biochemistry and history of sugar and his own journey to health. *Sweet Poison*, Penguin Books, London 2013

Nina Teicholz spent ten years investigating and debunking the myth that dietary fat is bad for us. A great read and a frightening revelation of bad science and prejudice. *The Big Fat Surprise: Why butter, meat and cheese belong in a healthy diet*, Scribe UK, 2015

Michael Moss talked to insiders from the food industry and reveals the greed and dirty tricks behind some of the biggest brands on the supermarket shelves. *Salt, Sugar, Fat: How the food giants hooked us*, WH Allen, London 2014

This interactive graphic from *British Medical Journal*, February 2015, is a remarkable revelation of the links between advisory bodies, academia and the food industry: www.bmj.com/content/350/bmj.h231/infographic

CONGRATULATIONS!

I want to congratulate you on your willingness to make a difference and your persistence in reading this book and working on each technique. You have started a huge and powerful change in your life. Keep using all the techniques. Even if you find some difficult and some easy, even if you think you don't need them, use them all as instructed and you will give yourself a massive boost to restore your own control of your appetite.

Remember, ... in control, you are free in relation to sugar. You ... or leave it. You will find that in everyday life you most ... partly because you know now the range of your ... d partly because your taste will readjust and ... that most of the time manufactured foods ta ... 'y too sweet and yet unsatisfying.

In your new life fresh ... and fresh water will be the basis of nourishment a... top of that you will add whatever types of food take your fancy.

I wish you a long, healthy and satisfying life!

Until we meet,

Paul McKenna
London 2016